Better Than Ever

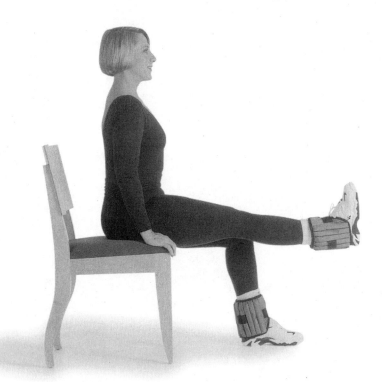

Better Than Ever

The 4-Week Workout Program for Women Over 40

**Lisa Hoffman, M.A.,
with Anita Weil Bell**

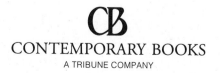

CONTEMPORARY BOOKS

A TRIBUNE COMPANY

Library of Congress Cataloging-in-Publication Data

Hoffman, Lisa.
    Better than ever : the 4-week workout program for women over 40 /
Lisa Hoffman, with Anita Weil Bell.
      p.   cm.
    Includes bibliographical references (p.).
    ISBN 0-8092-3123-9
    1. Exercise for women.   2. Middle aged women—Health and
hygiene.   I. Bell, Anita Weil.   II. Title.
   [RA778.H744   1997]
   613.7′1′082—dc20
                                    96-35398
                                       CIP

Cover design by Monica Baziuk
Cover photograph by Dorothy Handelman
Interior design based on one by Anne Chalmers
Interior photographs by Dorothy Handelman

Published by Contemporary Books
An imprint of NTC/Contemporary Publishing Company
Two Prudential Plaza, Chicago, Illinois 60601-6790
Manufactured in the United States of America
International Standard Book Number: 0-8092-3123-9
10   9   8   7   6   5   4   3   2   1

CONTENTS

ACKNOWLEDGMENTS

When I started Solo Fitness® in 1990, I truly thought it would be a solo endeavor. But as I began to explore the fitness concerns of midlife women, I realized the need to reach out to the dedicated health professionals working in this field. And when I decided to expand beyond one-on-one training and bring the information I had gathered to the public in a book, it became clear that this was not going to be a solo journey.

I thank the following people for their valuable help: Theresa Galsworthy, and the staff at the Hospital for Special Surgery, Osteoporosis Prevention Center in New York City, for spending time with an information hungry personal trainer, and for providing accessible, up-to-date resources and support; my professors at Columbia University Teachers College for insight into critical thinking and research and development; Carleen Lindsey, P.T., University of Connecticut Health Center, for expanding my knowledge of exercise for women with osteoporosis; and especially my cowriter, Anita Weil Bell, for her talent for turning my physiological exercise thoughts into reader-friendly English. Not only have we had a successful writing partnership, but we've also become friends and had a lot of laughs along the way. She has a true talent of understanding, discipline, and professionalism.

The authors thank the following people for giving their time and expertise to the book project:

- Sharon Akabas, Ph.D., Assistant Professor in Nutrition and Education, Columbia University Teachers College
- Richard Bockman, M.D., Ph.D., Professor of Medicine, Cornell University Medical Center; Head, Endocrine Service at the Hospital for Special Surgery, New York City
- Theresa Chiaia, P.T., Senior Physical Therapist, The Sports Medicine Center Hospital for Special Surgery, New York City
- Nancy Clark, M.S., R.D., Sports Nutritionist, Director of Nutri-

tion Services at Sports Medicine Brookline, Massachusetts

- Ronald DeMeersman, Ph.D., Professor of Applied Physiology, Columbia Teachers College
- Alice Domar, Ph.D., Assistant Professor of Medicine, Senior Scientist, Harvard Medical School, Mind/Body Institute
- William Evans, Ph.D., Director, Noll Physiological Research Center, Penn State University
- Theresa D. Galsworthy, R.N., O.N.C., Director of the Osteoporosis Prevention Center at the Hospital for Special Surgery, New York City
- Fredi Kronenberg, Ph.D., Director of Rosenthal Center for Alternative/Complementary Medicine, College of Physicians and Surgeons of Columbia University
- Lila Nachtigall, M.D., Professor of Obstetrics and Gynecology, New York University School of Medicine
- Elizabeth Lee Vliet, M.D., Founder, HER Place—The Woman's Center, Tucson, Arizona, and Fort Worth, Texas; Clinical Associate Professor, University of Arizona College of Medicine

For helping to make our photo shoot such a success, we thank Dorothy Handelman, our photographer, for her artistic vision and attention to detail; Revlon, Inc., for generously donating the services of makeup artist Harvey Helms and hair stylist Jamie Angel; Steven Gee for his hair styling; Reebok® International Ltd. for donating state-of-art sneakers and socks; K.D. dance® for the comfortable and attractive fitnesswear; Omni Fitness for contributing the weights and mat.

Much thanks and admiration to our fit and fabulous models (in order of appearance): Melissa Mittman, Yvonne Tatum, Faye Cone, Carol Levin, Janet Jacobs, Genia D'ambrosia, and Liina Broms.

Our gratitude to Gail Winston, Susan Schwartz, and our agents, Victoria Sanders and Faith Hamlin.

Lisa thanks the trainers who have worked with Solo Fitness® throughout the years, for their knowledge and assistance in enhancing the company; my clients, without whom this book would never have come to be —thank you for being the subjects of my fitness ideas and for always being honest about telling me what works and what doesn't in the real world of lifelong physical fitness; Sandy Chilewich for helping to put together the pieces of the photo shoot; Sarah Marks for her generous help and advice; Melissa Mittman for her valuable support from the beginning; Beth Klarreich and Paula Gifford for introducing me to personal training; my "Schwarzwald family," Dr. Claus and Meike Discher, Silke Fichter, and Dr. Andreas Schmid, for their long-distance friendship and helpful information; Mark Rapp for listening, troubleshooting, and caring along the way; my brother, Brian Hoffman, for keeping me focused and making sense of it all; and, most of all, my parents, Audrey and Harold Hoffman, for their neverending love and enthusiasm for my dreams and ambitions.

Anita thanks her husband, Jonathan Bell, and BlueBell, for their love and playfulness, and her family — Janet Jacobs, Laura Huennekens, and Shirley and Gilbert Weil, for all their love and positive energy.

INTRODUCTION

"I feel like I'm losing control," Sheryl said at our first personal training session. "I've gained weight, especially around the middle, although I'm not eating more than usual. I have trouble sleeping, and even when I do sleep well, I'm tired the next day. I can't concentrate at work and I get stressed out so easily. And now, on top of all this, my doctor says my cholesterol is high and I'm at risk for osteoporosis. I'm a busy woman. I can't afford to fall apart at age forty-nine!"

Sheryl was primarily motivated to start an exercise program because she was concerned about her risk of osteoporosis and heart disease. After several weeks of progress, however, she was delighted to discover that working out also relieved many of her menopausal symptoms.

By the second week of her exercise program, Sheryl experienced an upsurge in her energy level and felt focused and optimistic. By the third week she had lost weight and gained strength and flexibility. She was more confident about her body, which led to a rekindled interest in sex.

By the time Sheryl celebrated her fiftieth birthday, she felt stronger and leaner than she had in fifteen years. The results of her next physical examination were rewarding: Her cholesterol had dropped to a healthy level and she was maintaining bone density.

"The medical results are important," Sheryl told me, "But what's more important is how much better I feel every day. I tell all my friends who are worried about menopause: exercise! But a lot of them say they don't know how to get started or what type of exercise to do."

As the owner of Solo Fitness® and an exercise physiologist, I create exercise programs that are customized to the needs of midlife women. My goal in writing this book is to help you be your own personal trainer and feel better than ever. You'll learn all about different forms of aerobic exercise, strength-training workouts, and stretching for flexibility. Then you'll be ready to personalize the 4-Week Workout Program and enjoy safe, progressive fitness.

Since a healthy diet and a balanced lifestyle, in addition to exercise, are part of a woman's well-being, the program includes advice on nutrition, managing stress, and other issues. However, recommendations are not given here on hormone replacement therapy (HRT). This is a decision about which you need to educate yourself fully and consult with your physician. Whatever decision you make regarding HRT, you would be wise to include regular exercise as part of your health regime.

Perhaps you're approaching or going through menopause and you identify with some of Sheryl's symptoms. Maybe your doctor has said you have osteoporosis or are at risk for this disease. Or you're simply looking for a low-maintenance, low-cost, age-appropriate workout that's easy and fun to do. Whatever your needs or motivation, *Better Than Ever* offers a fitness routine that can fit into your busy life as a pleasure, not a chore.

The program meets the specific needs of midlife women by focusing on weight-bearing exercise. If "weight-bearing" sounds too serious, don't worry, it can be as simple as taking a walk through the park or doing a twenty-minute exercise session to your favorite music. To ensure that the program is safe and effective regardless of your experience, the strength-training routines have been designed with variations for different fitness levels. There is also a special strength workout for women with osteoporosis.

THE PROGRAM HAS THREE BASIC ELEMENTS

THE 4-WEEK WORKOUT PROGRAM: STRENGTH TRAINING ROUTINE — Twenty-minute strength-building and stretching routines you can do on your own at home.

AEROBIC ACTIVITIES — A menu for choosing aerobic forms you *enjoy*; guidelines for intensity, duration, and frequency.

LIFESTYLE LIFTS — Tips on nutrition, relaxation, and other ways to nurture your body and mind.

THE 4-WEEK WORKOUT PROGRAM WILL HELP YOU:

▶ Alleviate menopausal symptoms such as fatigue, moodiness, anxiety, depression, insomnia, weight gain, incontinence, and loss of interest in sex.

- ▸ Cope with hot flashes.
- ▸ Reduce your risk of osteoporosis and help maintain bone density.
- ▸ Reduce your risk of heart disease.
- ▸ Bring your weight to a healthy level and maintain it.
- ▸ Firm and tone your body.
- ▸ Increase your strength and muscle while you decrease body fat.
- ▸ Discover that exercise is fun and helps you feel better than ever.

Depending on your age, you may be wondering if you qualify as a midlife or menopausal woman. For the purposes of this program, "midlife" includes women ages forty to sixty. The term "menopausal" is used to refer to women who are in all three technical stages of menopause:

PERIMENOPAUSAL/PREMENOPAUSAL —the time during which a woman has experienced hormonal changes and/or irregularities in her menstrual cycle.

MENOPAUSE —a woman's final menstrual period.

POSTMENOPAUSAL —when a woman has not had a menstrual period for at least one year.

Basically, menopause means the end of menstruation and the cyclical ovarian process that began with puberty. The following chapters explain how exercise helps you through the physical and emotional changes of menopause and the health risks that may follow.

Midlife is a time when you deserve to enjoy a heightened sense of power, wisdom, independence, and self-acceptance. There's no reason why menopause should disrupt your life and mark the beginning of physical decline. Instead, it can be a turning point that inspires you to start and stay with a fitness program that makes you feel better than ever. *Better Than Ever: The 4-Week Workout Program for Women Over 40* will help you regain and retain all the strength, energy, and confidence you need to enjoy an active and satisfying future.

Better Than Ever

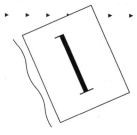

TAKING CONTROL: HOW EXERCISE HELPS THE MOOD SWINGS OF MENOPAUSE

"Exercise tends to improve mood and sense of well-being through enhancing endorphins and other chemical messengers in the brain as well as through the improved sense of self-esteem with the accomplishment."

—ELIZABETH LEE VLIET, M.D.

Founder, HER Place—
The Woman's Center, Tucson,
Arizona, and Fort Worth, Texas

One of the most frequent concerns I hear from women who are going through menopause is: "I feel like I'm losing control over my body, and even my life." After a month of regular exercise, these same women report: "It helps me feel in control." One woman said, "It lets me be in control when all these uncontrollable forces are taking over my body."

As a midlife woman, you've probably achieved a great deal in your personal and professional life—and it hasn't been easy! Then, just when you're ready to enjoy your hard-won rewards, a physical change starts to disrupt your life. It's enough to throw any woman off balance.

Exercising is a wonderfully effective way to regain a sense of control. On the physical side, working out helps you manage your weight and body shape, and develop strength and power. On the emotional/psychological side, sticking with an exercise program gives you a feeling of accomplishment and commitment you can apply to any aspect of your life.

This is not about being a control freak. We all need as much spontaneity and humor in our lives as possible. And we all know there is a certain element of chance in life. What exercise offers is a healthy, *balanced* sense of being in control.

The key to enjoying this benefit is to have an organized exercise program you do on a continual basis. Working out erratically won't give you any sense of control, and it won't control the symptoms of menopause. The satisfaction and benefits result from a steady routine.

That's where the 4-Week Workout Program comes to the rescue. The program provides a structure you can fit into your own schedule and lifestyle. You'll know exactly what you need to do and when you need to do it. You'll be in control of this important area of your life.

ENDORPHINS: THE NATURAL HIGH

Does it sometimes seem that all life's pleasures have risks and side effects nowadays? Eating delicious foods, sunbathing, sex . . . isn't there anything safe and guilt-free anymore? The answer is, yes; there's moderate exercise, a way to feel great and enjoy yourself with only *positive* side effects!

We've all heard about "runner's high," but a more accurate term for this phenomenon would be "exercise euphoria," since any type of sustained aerobic exercise can produce this sensation. And exercise euphoria is not just a vague feeling, it stems from a physiological response. Here's how it works:

Exercise stimulates the production of endorphins, which are neurotransmitters released by the pituitary gland. These clever chemicals induce a feeling of euphoria and also alter nerve transmission in a manner that lessens pain.

Studies have shown that vigorous workouts can increase endorphin levels by as much as five hundred percent. This helps create a feeling of well-being and is a valuable tool in overcoming the blues and the depression that can accompany menopause.

EXERCISE TO BEAT THE BLUES

According to a 1994 *Prevention* magazine poll of 2,000 women, 26 percent experience some depression when going through menopause. There are many complex physical, chemical, emotional, and societal reasons for this increase in the incidence of depression. Exercise helps in a number of ways.

On the chemical side, sustained exercise increases the production of endorphins, which often lifts the spirits. On the physical side, exercise improves posture, which can uplift the mood as well as the spine. Physical activity can also aid weight loss, which often raises a woman's mood along with her self-esteem.

Psychologically, exercise helps women overcome the depressing (and wrong!) idea that menopause signals the beginning of the end.

Instead, it can be a period of rejuvenation and the beginning of a satisfying new stage of life.

Elaine, a real estate agent, found herself sinking into a depression when her periods became erratic at age forty-eight. "I felt like I was going to lose my looks, lose my energy, and turn into an old lady. I just couldn't stop the negative thoughts. A down attitude is disastrous in my line of work, and it was really affecting my sales. I went to a therapist, and it helped to talk, but I still felt depressed.

"What saved me was that my sister insisted I start going to her gym for step classes. It was amazing how the classes made me feel more optimistic and positive. Now I go three or four times a week and it never fails to lift me up. By the end of a class, I feel like I can handle anything."

There are many degrees and types of depression, and exercise is certainly not a panacea for everyone. If depression is affecting your ability to function, professional support is needed. But for many cases of mild midlife depression, exercise can have a dramatic effect. It also helps the flip-side of depression: anxiety, irritability, and tension.

EXERCISE AS A DE-STRESSER

▸ ▸ ▸ ▸ ▸ ▸ ▸ ▸ ▸ ▸ ▸

Some women report that menopause feels like an endless bout of PMS. According to a 1991 Gallup poll of 705 women, three in five report anxiety, irritability, and nervousness as symptoms of menopause. The fluctuation of hormones and hot flashes coupled with the larger issues of aging and sexuality are enough to put any woman on edge.

Exercise, along with relaxation techniques you'll do as part of the program, is the safest and surest way to control anxiety. The influence of exercise on mood swings illustrates that the mind and body are interconnected. The concentration and control it takes to work out, coupled with the increase in heart rate and circulation, is stimulating and relaxing at the same time. Your body revs up and your mind calms down.

Evie, who has a demanding customer relations job, had a habit of having two or three glasses of wine after work to relax. But as she approached menopause, she found the wine was exacerbating her hot flashes and fatigue. She had to find another way to reduce stress.

"Actually it was my dog that gave me the solution. He's always raring to go when I get home. So instead of taking him for a ten-minute walk, I decided to start taking him on longer walks. That way I could get my exercise and get over my guilt at leaving him alone all day.

"I found that after about fifteen minutes of brisk walking I really began to relax and get into a better frame of mind. Now we walk for thirty or forty minutes almost every day and I skip the wine. I feel so relaxed afterwards, ready to forget about work and enjoy my evening."

There's another bonus to exercising for stress reduction. People with well-conditioned hearts are better able to withstand the physical effects of stress. They are able to maintain lower heart rates under stress, and are more likely to remain calm and in control.

Exercise is both a stimulant and a tranquilizer. It's one of the few ways to cope with mood swings that has beneficial side effects . . . and it's cheaper than a shopping spree!

EXERCISE FOR THE PROFESSIONAL ADVANTAGE

▶ ▶ ▶ ▶ ▶ ▶ ▶ ▶ ▶ ▶ ▶

Many women find that menopause disrupts their work. Dragging through the day after a sleepless night, hot flashes in the middle of a meeting, skirts that are suddenly too tight around the middle—who needs any of it?

Exercise is a highly successful method of easing the pressures menopause can exert on your work life. Physical activity helps you sleep well so you're rested and ready to handle your responsibilities. It alleviates anxiety and irritability. It boosts energy, builds confidence, and enhances self-image.

I asked my clients, all midlife women, how their exercise programs have helped them in their careers. Here are some of the responses.

A stockbroker said: "In my line I can't afford to lose speed. I have to have as much push and energy as the twenty-five-year-old just starting out. Weight training and the treadmill help me keep my edge."

An advertising account executive said: "It sounds silly, but now when I'm making a presentation I can concentrate on the work and not worry about my butt sticking out or my jacket looking too tight. I can focus on my audience and not my body."

A children's clothing designer said: "I find that exercise helps my creativity. Maybe it's the increased blood flow to the brain, but for some reason I get great ideas when I'm swimming."

Some women like to work out first thing in the morning, to start the day feeling energetic and accomplished. Others prefer to exercise after work to get rid of the tension of the day. Another option is to schedule a workout at lunchtime, a sure way to beat the afternoon slump.

Before starting the program, you'll review your lifestyle to decide when it's best to make your exercise appointments. Whatever schedule you choose, when you stick with it, you'll find that exercise has a positive effect on your work as well as your personal life.

EXERCISE

FOR ENERGY

Insomnia, fatigue, and lack of energy are major problems of menopause. According to the *Prevention* study, 41 percent of menopausal women report sleep problems and 37 percent feel fatigued. Yet most midlife women can't afford to slow down and are determined to maintain their busy lifestyles.

Exercise works in two ways to help women overcome fatigue. First, it often results in more restful sleep and alleviation of insomnia. Second, exercise actually *creates* more energy.

THE ENERGY MOLECULES

Almost everyone has experienced how a brisk walk or other physical activity washes away feelings of sluggishness. The physiological mechanism behind this miracle involves energy cells called adenosine triphosphate molecules (ATPs).

The energy in food is not transferred to cells directly; it is funneled through ATPs. The process of synthesizing food into these energy-rich cells is enhanced by sustained aerobic activity. In effect, aerobic exercise helps you produce a greater abundance of fuel for energy.

In addition to increasing the production of ATPs, exercise has a number of other fatigue-fighting benefits.

Cardiovascular exercise stimulates the heart to pump blood faster and increase circulation. This carries vital nutrients into the organs and muscles more efficiently, and sweeps away fatigue-causing substances. Exercise keeps the body balanced and the joints flexible, getting rid of that rusty feeling. It serves as a wake-up call to the nervous system, mobilizing the mind and body. It also raises the metabolic rate by increasing calorie expenditure.

The tricky part is to get yourself to exercise when you're feeling sluggish. The 4-Week Workout Program is designed to help you overcome this hurdle. Every week you'll make specific exercise appointments with yourself. You'll know exactly when you're going to exercise and what you're going to do, which makes it a whole lot easier to get up and do it. You'll be able to identify the optimal time to exercise and what form is best for you.

Angela, a fifty-one-year-old woman who works in publishing, had always experienced an afternoon slump that she fought with coffee. But as she reached menopause, she found that the slump had turned into serious fatigue, and that extra cups of coffee brought on hot flashes.

"I tried eating a light lunch, but even so I was absolutely exhausted by two o'clock. All I wanted to do was lie down and sleep, or cry. Finally a friend at work suggested that I join him on his lunchtime walks. He had started exercising after he had a scare with heart trouble.

"Now, instead of going out to the diner, I bring a light lunch to have at my desk, and then put on my sneakers and go for a half-hour walk. Even when it's raining, we're out there with our umbrellas. Everyone thinks we're crazy, but it really works. I come back feeling alert and alive and ready to work, instead of ready to drop."

OVERCOMING INSOMNIA

▸ ▸ ▸ ▸ ▸ ▸ ▸ ▸ ▸ ▸ ▸ ▸

"Hot flashes disturb sleep and sleep deprivation can cause anxiety and depression. Exercise tends to help people sleep better."

—ALICE DOMAR, PH.D.

Assistant Professor of Medicine, Harvard Medical School

Many women who previously had no trouble sleeping develop insomnia at menopause. The reasons include hot flashes that interrupt sleep, hormonal fluctuations, and increased stress and anxiety.

Exercise can help you sleep soundly by balancing and relaxing your body. It can reduce the muscle tension and emotional anxiety that exacerbate sleeplessness. As part of the 4-Week Workout Program you'll also learn relaxation techniques to help you sleep, sleep, sleep.

HOT FLASHES

▸ ▸ ▸ ▸ ▸ ▸ ▸ ▸ ▸ ▸ ▸

Since hot flashes are one of the most prevalent symptoms of menopause, you may wonder why I didn't start this book by proclaiming "Exercise eliminates hot flashes!" The reason is that it's not proven. All the benefits of exercise in this book are backed up by research and my own experience as a personal trainer and exercise physiologist. But the question of whether or not exercise reduces hot flashes is still debatable.

A study done at the University Hospital in Sweden indicates that exercise may have a positive effect. The researchers found that hot flashes were only half as common among the physically active women (21.5 percent) as in a control group of somewhat inactive women (48 percent). They concluded that these results could be due to exercise affecting one of the mechanisms that provokes hot flashes, involving neurotransmitter activity.

Exercise seems to help some but not all women with hot flashes. Overall health, nutrition, genetics, and just plain luck are also part of the hot flash equation.

Many women notice a drop in the number of hot flashes after starting their exercise programs. Others report no change in the frequency, but do find that they are able to cope with the hot flashes better. More confidence and less overall anxiety as a result of exercising makes it easier to deal with this symptom.

Another way in which the 4-Week Workout Program is likely to help is through dietary changes. Alcohol and caffeine can trigger hot flashes, and cutting down on these is part of the program. Several studies have also indicated that relaxation techniques can diminish the frequency of hot flashes.

At any rate, when you're feeling good about yourself, looking fit and confident, and pumping endorphins, you're more likely to react to hot flashes with a shrug and a healthy sense of humor.

CELEBRATE YOURSELF: BODY IMAGE AND SEXUALITY

"I'm eating the same as I always did, but I'm gaining weight!" This is a familiar lament among midlife women. And with menopause many women experience a sudden thickening around the waist, loss of muscle tone and skin tone, and extra pounds on the scale.

The first question many clients ask at their training consultation is the one you may have in mind: "Will I lose weight on this program?" The answer is a definite maybe. It depends on many factors: diet, genetics, and your current physical state.

In other words, if you're a perfectly healthy weight but don't look like a runway model, you are not likely to lose many pounds on the 4-Week Workout Program. But if you are overweight, and you follow the dietary suggestions as well as the exercise routines, you *are* likely to slim down.

Diet and genetics, along with exercise, are key components in weight loss and maintenance. For example, if you choose to do the exercise part of the program and continue eating fatty foods, you may tone up without actually losing pounds. If you have a genetic predisposition toward being a large woman, the program will help you become firm and flexible but not necessarily thin.

What really matters is not the number on the scale, it's your health and body image. *Don't be a slave to the scale.* Life is about being a healthy, vital, loving, positive person. What counts is that you're active and you live your life to the fullest.

We've all known skinny women who never think they're thin enough. And we've all marveled at big women who are self-confident, active, and attractive. What's the difference and what's the secret? It's *body image.* When you're comfortable and proud of your body you project confidence and exude natural appeal.

This is where exercise works its magic. When you exercise regularly, gradually building up your endurance and strength, you learn to respect your body. As you progress and achieve new stages of fitness, you learn to love your body and develop the innate self-confidence that is one of the secrets of attraction.

When women reach menopause, they often feel as if their sexuality and beauty are waning. This can lead to anxiety, depression, and problems in relationships.

The antidote to this negative mindset is physical activity. Exercise has an almost magical ability to make you feel good about your body. It's the best way to shake off ageist, sexist, defeatist prejudices about mature women. Exercise makes you feel strong, confident, attractive, and energetic—all the qualities that are typically associated with youth, but rightfully belong to *all* women.

FEELING BETTER, LOOKING BETTER

▶ ▶ ▶ ▶ ▶ ▶ ▶ ▶ ▶ ▶

The enhanced body image that comes with regular exercise is based on reality. With the 4-Week Workout Program, you will improve your physical appearance as well as your body image. Here's how it works.

BETTER POSTURE The strength-training and flexibility exercises will improve your posture, enabling you to look taller and slimmer without dieting or wearing high heels.

MUSCLE TONE The 4-Week Workouts will help you develop toned muscles. You'll gain an enhanced sense of confidence and independence along with stronger muscles.

CONTOURS, NOT BULK When women hear the words "strength training" they sometimes worry about looking like female bodybuilders. And while these athletes certainly have their appeal, not all of us are comfortable with that degree of muscle development.

Let me reassure you: If you follow the program, you'll shape and contour your body and may build moderate muscles, but you won't be ready for the Miss Olympia contest. Female bodybuilders work out for many, many hours a day, using heavy weights to reach this degree of development.

LOSE FAT, GAIN MUSCLE   Sometimes women drop to a smaller size when they start exercising regularly, but their weight remains the same on the scale. This is because muscle weighs more than fat. It also looks a lot more attractive.

I suggest that you don't even get on the scale for the first two weeks of the program. The scale is irrelevant since you can lose fat and gain muscle without losing a pound. But you'll notice the difference, and so will everyone else.

EXERCISE AS AN APHRODISIAC

▸ ▸ ▸ ▸ ▸ ▸ ▸ ▸ ▸ ▸ ▸

Maria, who has enjoyed a good marriage for over twenty-five years, found the most distressing symptom of menopause was her diminished interest in sex. "I've always been very sexual. But when I stopped getting my periods I just lost my desire. Partly it was physical, that dry feeling. But I know it was also in my head. I just didn't feel desirable anymore."

Although the decline in estrogen has a physical affect on sexuality, these physical symptoms can usually be managed. Yet beyond the hormonal changes lies a stronger enemy of sexuality: the societal and emotional implications of menopause.

In a society that puts such a high premium on youth, it's difficult for many women to maintain their sexual self-esteem after menopause. With movies, TV shows, and advertising focusing on young lust, it's hard to find role models of mature sexuality. In addition, some women remember their mothers or grandmothers as being "past all that" sexually when they were in their fifties.

The good news is that these stereotypes are rapidly changing. Today's midlife women are certainly not ready to retire to the rocker and let young people have all the fun.

The media is slowly beginning to feature sexy midlife women in romantic situations. And this change is due in large part to the fitness revolution. As more women stay physically fit after menopause, they are changing the image of the mature woman.

Since fitness is an integral part of sexuality, exercise can help revive desire. Maria started taking a dance exercise class because there was incidence of heart disease in her family and she was concerned about her cardiovascular fitness. But she found the workouts pumped up more than her heart.

"After my second dance class, I felt all limber and full of energy. I had fantasies about being a Broadway dancer. So I dug out my old fishnet stockings. I felt like making love for the first time in months. Boy, was my husband in for a pleasant surprise!"

Exercise enhances midlife sexuality in many ways. It improves body image so you feel more confident in bed. By increasing circulation, a vigorous workout can make your skin feel more sensitive and sensual. It helps you overcome fatigue and have the energy for lovemaking. And it improves your posture, body contours, and muscle tone so you look and feel more attractive.

"I really tightened everything up with my dancing," says Maria. "And now my husband says I look better than when we first got married. Hearing that sure is a turn-on!"

THE KEGEL EXERCISES

The Kegel exercises, which you'll learn to do as part of the program, have a dual purpose: they can lead to a more intense feeling of sexual stimulation, and they help eliminate the problem of stress incontinence.

Stress incontinence, or occasional loss of bladder control, is an embarrassing condition that some women experience with the onset of menopause. The Kegel exercises, developed by Dr. Arnold Kegel at UCLA, can be a tremendous help.

"Kegels," as they are called, are simple exercises that involve contracting and releasing the vaginal muscles. They are the same exercises as those recommended during pregnancy. In addition to relieving incontinence, they can help keep the pelvic organs healthy and increase sexual pleasure.

In addition to doing Kegel exercises as part of the program, you can easily incorporate them into your day. You can do these private exercises at your desk, in your car, or wherever you please. And this little secret can help you enjoy a long lifetime of sexual fitness.

EXERCISE AND OSTEOPOROSIS

Osteoporosis is a condition in which a loss of bone tissue causes bones to become porous and fragile. Along with a loss in bone strength, people with osteoporosis experience a vulnerability to bone fractures. It is a major health problem, affecting more than 20 million women and 5 million men in the United States. The condition causes approximately 1.5 million hip, spine, and wrist fractures each year at an estimated cost of over 10 billion dollars.

Since the risk of osteoporosis dramatically increases after menopause, this disease is of major concern to midlife women. According to the National Osteoporosis Foundation, women are four times more likely to develop the disease than men, and one-third of American women over age fifty will eventually have a fracture due to this condition.

There are two categories of osteoporosis: primary (Type I) and secondary (Type II). Secondary or Type II osteoporosis, which occurs in both men and women age seventy and older, is associated with aging and may be caused by age-related processes. Primary or Type I osteoporosis, which is the category we'll be discussing, is far more common in women. Type I characteristically occurs within fifteen to twenty years after menopause, and is caused in part by rapid bone loss due to the sharp decline in estrogen.

A balanced exercise program plays an integral role in helping to prevent osteoporosis and in reducing the risk of fractures in women who have been diagnosed. To understand the impact of exercise, it's helpful to have a basic knowledge of the physiology of bone.

THE BASICS OF BONE
▸ ▸ ▸ ▸ ▸ ▸ ▸ ▸ ▸ ▸ ▸

Bone is living, growing tissue that is constantly being renewed. In this ongoing process, old bone is removed and new bone is formed by the production of a soft protein framework (mostly collagen) which hardens when the mineral calcium phosphate is deposited.

There are two types of bone: trabecular and cortical. Trabecular bone comprises the porous interior of the bone. With a texture similar to a honeycomb, it acts as a cushion and a reservoir for calcium. Cortical bone is the dense outer portion of the bone. It offers maximum protection and strength, and accounts for 80 percent of total bone tissue.

Both types of bone are found throughout the body in varying proportions. The vertebrae and ends of the long arm and leg bones contain the highest percentage of trabecular bone. Since the bone loss of osteoporosis occurs most rapidly in trabecular bone, these areas of the hip, spine, and wrist become the most vulnerable.

Bone remodeling is the two-stage process by which bone renews itself. In the first stage, resorption, bone cells called osteoclasts dissolve bone tissue on the surface, creating a small cavity. In the second stage, formation, cells called osteoblasts fill in the cavities with new bone. The remodeling process can be activated by chemical factors such as hormones and calcium, or physical influences such as exercise and gravity. Bone remodeling is more rapid in trabecular than cortical bone. There is eight times more turnover in trabecular bone than in cortical.

During childhood and adolescence, new bone is added to the skeleton faster than old bone is removed, allowing the bones to become larger and heavier. Between the ages of twenty-five and thirty-five most people reach peak bone mass (maximum bone density and strength). After age thirty-five, approximately, bone removal begins to overtake bone replacement in both men and women. For this reason, the ideal time to begin osteoporosis prevention is in childhood. If you have daughters or granddaughters, you can help by encouraging them to consume calcium-rich foods and exercise.

Adequate calcium intake and regular exercise throughout the growing years are believed to protect against fractures in later life. The more bone mass a person deposits in their bone "bank account," the more withdrawals they can tolerate in later years without developing dangerously low bone density.

In women the process of bone loss accelerates after menopause. Experts believe this loss is mainly due to the decline in the production of estrogen, a hormone produced primarily by the ovaries. Estrogen has a protective effect on bone that is lost at menopause. The risk or condition of osteoporosis is one of the primary reasons some physicians advise their patients to go on hormone replacement therapy (HRT) or other nonhormonal medications.

WHO IS AT RISK
FOR OSTEOPOROSIS?
▶ ▶ ▶ ▶ ▶ ▶ ▶ ▶ ▶ ▶

Everyone who ages loses bone, but not everyone develops osteoporosis. A variety of factors, some controllable and some not, determine who is at risk. These are the major risk factors:

GENDER Women can lose up to 20 percent of their total bone mass in the first five to seven years after menopause. It's critical that women take steps to protect their bone during these first postmenopausal years.

AGE The longer a person lives, the more her or his chance of developing osteoporosis increases. However, the rapid bone loss of osteoporosis does not have to be a normal or inevitable part of aging.

LACK OF PHYSICAL ACTIVITY People who are inactive or bedridden are at higher risk for osteoporosis. Weight-bearing exercise is a powerful tool for preventing bone loss.

LACK OF CALCIUM Adequate calcium intake is essential to building and maintaining strong, healthy bones.

THIN, SMALL-FRAMED BODY Petite women generally have less bone to spare than big-boned women. Very thin women are at greater risk for fractures due to the lesser amount of weight being exerted on the bones.

RACE Caucasian and Asian women are at higher risk of developing osteoporosis than African-Americans.

PREMATURE MENOPAUSE Women who experience surgical or naturally occurring premature menopause lose the protective effects of estrogen at an earlier age.

ANOREXIA AND OVERTRAINING Decreased estrogen, indicated by irregular menstruation, can also be caused by anorexia, intense dieting, or overexercising. This is the female athlete triad. Many athletes and ballet dancers experience amenorrhea (cessation of menstruation) and resulting bone loss due to estrogen deficiency.

HEREDITY Reduced bone mass and susceptibility to fractures may be influenced by heredity.

CIGARETTE SMOKING AND EXCESSIVE CAFFEINE OR ALCOHOL CONSUMPTION Smoking is damaging to bones. Drinking caffeinated or alcoholic beverages in excess is also a risk.

CERTAIN MEDICATIONS Long-term, high-dosage use of gluco-corticoids (anti-inflammatories used to treat asthma, arthritis, and some cancers) can lead to bone tissue loss. High dosages of anti-seizure drugs cause less calcium to be available for bone remodeling. Bone loss can also result from excessive thyroid hormone, diuretics (excluding thiazides), and heparin use.

HOW TO DETERMINE YOUR RISK OF OSTEOPOROSIS

▶ ▶ ▶ ▶ ▶ ▶ ▶ ▶ ▶ ▶ ▶

Osteoporosis has been called a silent disease because often no symptoms appear until a fracture occurs. Women may not know they have osteoporosis until their bones become so weak that a sudden strain, bump, or fall causes a fracture or reveals a seriously deteriorated vertebra.

Early prevention and detection of osteoporosis are key elements in preventing fractures. The goal is to identify women with low bone mass in enough time to prevent fractures from occurring.

To find out if you're at risk for osteoporosis, it is useful to check the list of risk factors, but it's not enough. The only way to be sure about your bone condition is through medical tests that measure bone mineral content in various sites.

The different types of bone density tests include single photon absorptiometry (SPA), which measures the forearm; and dual photon absorptiometry (DPA) and dual-energy x-ray absorptiometry (DEXA), both of which measure the hip and spine. Quantitative computed tomography (QCAT scan) is another procedure which does a series of cross-sectional images of the body. These tests are generally safe and painless, and are available in hospital and clinical settings. In addition, biochemical markers of bone remodeling can allow determination of the *rate* of bone turnover. This is usually done with a urine test. Medical insurance may cover the costs of the tests, depending on the plan.

It is recommended that most menopausal women, regardless of risk factors, have a baseline bone density test. This enables you to assess your risk of fracture and take steps to prevent further bone loss. It is useful information for selecting the safest form of aerobic exercise and the appropriate strength-training workout.

The data from the bone density test will help your physician assess your bone health and risk of future fractures. There are three basic outcomes of the tests:

▶ A healthy bone mass level
▶ A condition of osteopenia, which is low bone density that can result in osteoporosis
▶ A condition of osteoporosis

According to the World Health Organization (WHO) and the International Society for Clinical Densitometry, osteoporosis is defined as

2.5 standard deviations (SD) or more below the young normal peak bone mass; while osteopenia is defined as a deviation of more than 1.0 SD below the young adult mean but less than 2.5 SD below this value.

If you have osteopenia or osteoporosis, your physician may recommend hormone replacement therapy (HRT), which consists of estrogen and progesterone. Estrogen is one of the most common drugs prescribed for mature women and has been the mainstay of osteoporosis treatment in the United States and much of Europe over the past decade.

There are also several nonhormonal options for drug treatment of osteoporosis. Alendronate sodium was approved by the F.D.A. (Food and Drug Administration) in October 1995. It works by inhibiting bone resorption or breakdown. The most common mild side effects reported are nausea, heartburn, gas, and abdominal pain.

Calcitonin is available as injectable salmon calcitonin or an intranasal formulation. It works by suppressing bone resorption in women with elevated turnover.

Slow-release sodium fluoride is another nonhormonal method of treating osteoporosis. To date, a medical advisory committee to the F.D.A. has recommended regulatory approval and other treatments are on the horizon. Studies have shown a decrease of spine fractures in those with mild to moderate osteopenia, and this method may help prevent the first fracture.

Your doctor should also discuss the important lifestyle components of managing osteoporosis:

- Nutritional status and calcium intake
- Exercise
- Awareness of posture in daily living
- Accident-proofing your environment

This book focuses on the role of exercise in managing osteoporosis and preventing fractures. But please be aware that exercise is an *adjunct* to a comprehensive program for osteoporosis, which should be guided by a knowledgeable health care provider.

EXERCISE AND OSTEOPOROSIS

▸ ▸ ▸ ▸ ▸ ▸ ▸ ▸ ▸ ▸ ▸

In 1892 a German medical researcher observed that bone architecture was influenced by mechanical stresses. This led to the development of Wolff's Law, which states that bone remodeling is directly dependent on the mechanical load placed upon it.

Bone responds to the work your muscle places on it. For example, in a bicep curl, the shortening and lengthening of a muscle while moving a weight works the muscle. This, in turn, places stress on the bone. Weight-bearing exercise compresses and bends the long bones, increasing bone mineral content, thus strengthening bone.

To work bone you have to work muscle. And the bone that benefits is the one related to the specific muscle you work. The bone benefits of exercise are site specific. This is one reason why it's necessary to have a balanced exercise program that works all the muscles.

Nearly a century after the formulation of Wolff's Law, the National Institutes of Health recognized this principle in practical terms at their 1984 Health Consensus Development Conference on Osteoporosis. At this pivotal conference, the NIH officially recommended exercise for the prevention and treatment of osteoporosis.

A number of research studies have confirmed that exercise can help build bone mass in younger women and build or maintain bone mass in postmenopausal women.

In 1994 a study was conducted at the USDA Human Nutrition Research Center on Aging (HNRCA) at Tufts University by a team of researchers that included William Evans, Ph.D. The subjects were forty postmenopausal women between the ages of fifty and seventy. The women, who were sedentary and estrogen-depleted, were advised to increase their calcium intake to at least 800 mg a day in addition to exercising.

Their exercise regime consisted of a forty-five-minute high-intensity strength-training session (with five different exercises) twice a week for one year. After a year, tests showed an overall increase in the femoral neck bone and lumbar spine bone mineral density of the women who participated in the strength training and a decrease in the control group, who did not exercise or increase their calcium intake. Muscle mass, muscle strength, and dynamic balance also increased in the exercising women and decreased in the control.

Dr. Evans explains: "Resistance training has a major effect on bone health, not just in the lumbar spine but in the proximal femur (hip), lower back, and total skeleton.

"In addition, unlike any other intervention strategy for bone health, exercise has an effect on the other risk factors for osteoporotic fracture. Exercise can also improve balance, strength, increase levels of physical activity, and increase muscle mass. Virtually all of the risk factors are affected by strength training."

An earlier study led by Gail Dalsky, Ph.D., (then at the Washington University School of Medicine) in 1988 involved thirty-five healthy, sedentary, postmenopausal women. The women were given 1,500 mg of calcium daily and participated in an aerobic exercise program. Their exercise consisted of walking, jogging, and stair climbing at 70 to 90 percent of maximal oxygen uptake capacity for fifty to sixty minutes, three times weekly—a very vigorous program.

After nine months, bone mineral content increased 5.2 percent above the baseline in the exercising women, while there was little change (−1.4 percent) in the control group. After twenty-two months, the total change in bone mineral content for the exercising group was +6.1 percent above baseline. Thirteen months after the women stopped training, their bone mass had reverted back to baseline levels. This is further evidence of the need for continuing regular exercise to maintain bone health.

Other studies have been less conclusive on the ability of exercise to *increase* bone mass in postmenopausal women. However, it is generally accepted that exercise, combined with adequate calcium intake, can help slow the loss of bone. It also builds greater stability to reduce the chance of falls and fractures in women who are at risk.

THE RIGHT EXERCISE FOR WOMEN WITH OSTEOPOROSIS

▸ ▸ ▸ ▸ ▸ ▸ ▸ ▸ ▸ ▸ ▸

While there is yet no specific exercise prescription for osteoporosis, the overall recommendation is to engage in weight-bearing aerobic exercise for at least thirty minutes three or more days a week, and two sessions of strength training per week. Weight-bearing exercise involves aerobic activities that are performed while standing.

In Chapter 17 you'll find guidelines for women with osteoporosis on the frequency, intensity, and duration of recommended aerobic activities. You'll also find a strength workout especially designed to meet the needs of women with osteopenia or osteoporosis. This workout can be done throughout the four weeks of the Workout Program for Women Over 40, in place of the other strength workouts.

If you have been diagnosed with osteopenia or osteoporosis, you need to consult with your health professional before starting this or any exercise program. Since this condition has widely varying degrees of severity, you may need to modify your activity.

In general, there are certain exercise precautions for women with osteoporosis:

▸ No forward flexion (bending forward)
▸ No twisting movements
▸ No high-impact activity
▸ Be careful while moving in and out of positions during exercise

Despite a few restrictions, there is a wide range of enjoyable exercise options available for women with bone conditions. Exercise can give you an opportunity to expand your life at a time when osteoporosis may be limiting. It can replace pain and fear with confidence and joy in movement.

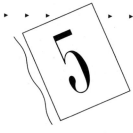

5

EXERCISE FOR A
HEALTHY HEART

"The positive influence of exercise on cardiovascular health is multifactorial. The bottom line is that exercise has a cardioprotective effect."

— RONALD DE MEERSMAN, PH.D.

Many people are unaware that heart disease is the leading cause of death for American women as well as men. There is a general misconception that women are somewhat immune to this disease. But nearly half of the approximately 500,000 Americans who die of heart attacks each year are female.

Although women lag ten years behind men in developing heart disease, after the age of sixty-five, women's risk of heart attack is nearly as high as men's. In addition, the survival rate for women with heart disease is significantly lower than it is for men.

The myth that women are not as vulnerable as men to heart disease stems from the protective effect of estrogen. However, since the risk of heart disease can rise sharply after menopause, heart disease is a primary health concern for midlife women. Women, as much as men, need to protect their heart and artery health through good nutrition and exercise.

THE HUMAN HEART

To understand what causes cardiovascular disease, it's helpful to understand the working of a healthy heart. In a well-functioning system, blood is collected by the veins and taken into the right atrium, a chamber of the heart. It then enters the right ventricle, which serves as a pumping chamber. Contractions force this blood into the lungs, where it acquires a fresh load of oxygen.

The blood flows from the lungs to the left atrium, which pumps it into the left ventricle. The left ventricle, known as the powerhouse of the heart, pumps blood into the arterial system through the aorta, which is the largest artery in the body.

The hardworking muscles of the left ventricle relax and contract about sixty times a minute, twenty-four hours a day. To keep this miraculous system going, the heart needs a constant supply of arterial blood, which it obtains from the aorta through the right and left coronary arteries. These two arteries are wrapped around the exterior of the heart, and are constantly moved by the vigorous motion of the heart wall.

It is these coronary arteries that are involved in heart attacks (also called massive coronaries or myocardial infarctions). Attacks can result when the coronary arteries are clogged and unable to deliver fresh blood to the walls of the heart. When this occurs, part of the heart actually dies. In a sense, heart disease is artery disease that affects the heart muscle.

THE ROLE OF CHOLESTEROL
▶ ▶ ▶ ▶ ▶ ▶ ▶ ▶ ▶ ▶ ▶

Healthy arterial blood is a thin fluid without excess fat or cholesterol. It moves easily through the blood vessels into the tissues, carrying oxygen and nutrients to all the body's muscles, skin, and organs, including the heart.

Fat and cholesterol in the bloodstream turn the blood into a heavier substance that is more difficult for the heart to push through the arteries and into the smaller blood vessels. Excess cholesterol obstructions in the arteries cause the heart to work even harder, and can end up blocking the blood supply and contributing to a heart attack.

A certain amount of cholesterol is produced by the body to perform a number of functions. This form of cholesterol is a waxy noncaloric substance involved with the production of sex hormones and adrenal hormones, and the synthesis of bile for digestive purposes. It is carried along with fat and protein in the bloodstream.

The body produces sufficient cholesterol to do its assigned jobs. *Excess* cholesterol, the type that causes trouble, is ingested through animal foods: dairy products, eggs, and red meat, and fish and poultry to a lesser degree. All animal foods contain some cholesterol, while all vegetable foods contain none.

It is the cholesterol that is ingested which elevates the blood cholesterol above the safe range of 200 mg/dL or less. Excess cholesterol in the blood is attracted to already damaged cells in the walls of the arteries. While a certain amount of damage is inevitable, additional injury to the arterial walls is caused by the presence of fat, oil, carbon monoxide from smoking, and other factors. Excess cholesterol intermingles with the cells of the arterial lining, creating a swelling around the injured cells. This swelling is known as cholesterol plaque.

As long as there is excess cholesterol in the blood, these lumps continue to build, causing a hardening and narrowing of the arteries (atherosclerosis). This results in a loss of arterial compliance, the process by which the arteries help the blood move through the body. It forces the heart to work harder and lessens the supply of oxygenated blood to body cells beyond the congested point. The end result can be a coronary heart attack.

The *type* of cholesterol in the blood, not just the level, is critical in cardiovascular health. There are several types of lipoproteins, or carriers of cholesterol, and also subsets of these lipoproteins.

HDL (high-density lipoprotein) is known as the "good" cholesterol because it moves the cholesterol out of the arteries and into the liver, where it is converted into bile and excreted. People with high levels of HDL cholesterol have a reduced risk of heart disease.

LDL (low-density lipoprotein) is a dangerous type of cholesterol that builds up in the walls of the arteries and creates blockages. A diet high in animal fat creates higher levels of LDL cholesterol, while a diet low in animal foods leads to a lower level.

ESTROGEN AND HEART DISEASE

▸ ▸ ▸ ▸ ▸ ▸ ▸ ▸ ▸ ▸ ▸

Estrogen, one of the two major female hormones, helps to protect premenopausal women from narrowing of the arteries and heart attack. While researchers are still working to identify the exact mechanism of this protective effect, it is known that estrogen has a positive influence on blood cholesterol by raising the HDL level and lowering the LDL level. Some experts believe estrogen is also involved in lowering blood pressure, a contributing factor in heart health.

When estrogen production declines at menopause, women lose its protective effect. This is one of the primary reasons why many physicians advise their patients to go on HRT.

A large-scale research program conducted at Harvard University involving 32,000 nurses indicated that women who took estrogen had 50 percent fewer heart attacks than those who did not. Yet despite these and other results, the use of ERT (estrogen replacement therapy) or HRT as preventive medicine is still being studied.

One of the chief concerns involves the possibility of an increased risk of cancer due to ERT, particularly cancers of the breast, uterus, and endometrium. Many doctors now prescribe taking progesterone with estrogen to offset this danger.

It is not yet known whether estrogen taken in combination with progestin retains its cardioprotective effect. However, results of a study by the NIH, called the Postmenopausal Estrogen-Progestin Intervention Trial (PEPI), indicate continued benefits with HRT.

The issue of hormone therapy for protection against heart disease is complex and controversial. Ultimately, it is a personal choice that should be made after you educate yourself thoroughly and weigh the pros and cons. But regardless of what you decide regarding hormone therapy, one fact is crystal clear: Exercise is essential for protecting your heart.

HEART DISEASE RISK FACTORS FOR WOMEN

▸ ▸ ▸ ▸ ▸ ▸ ▸ ▸ ▸ ▸

The loss of protective estrogen at menopause is a primary risk factor for heart disease among women, along with advancing age. Yet since many women live long lives with healthy hearts, it's worthwhile to examine the many risk factors that can be controlled through lifestyle choices. Once you are aware of these factors, you'll be motivated to make the changes you need to reduce your risk.

A SEDENTARY LIFESTYLE In 1992 the American Heart Association (AHA) declared lack of exercise to be a major risk factor for heart disease, as significant as smoking, high cholesterol, and high blood pressure. The association had long said that inactivity raises risk, but found recently that scientific evidence had grown strong enough to list lack of exercise as a *major* risk factor. The AHA stated that even modest physical activity could lower a sedentary person's risk of heart disease.

HIGH FAT CONSUMPTION A diet high in animal fats can damage arteries and lead to a high cholesterol level, a major risk factor. Women who eat mostly low-cholesterol foods can reduce their risk of heart attack by as much as one-third.

OBESITY Women who are more than 20 percent above the recommended weight for their height have an elevated risk of heart disease. Fat is particularly dangerous when it is distributed around the abdomen and stomach (visceral fat) rather than the hips and thighs. Reducing dietary fat and increasing exercise can help control this problem.

CIGARETTE SMOKING The Surgeon General's office has estimated that up to 40 percent of all deaths from coronary artery disease are directly attributable to smoking. A study of 1,000 nurses found that even women who smoke as little as one to four cigarettes a day had a risk two to three times greater than nonsmoking women. In addition, smoking can advance the onset of menopause by about five years, adding the risk factor of estrogen deficiency. The hopeful news is that a woman's heart disease risk can drop to normal as quickly as two to three years after she quits smoking, depending on her age and the extent of her smoking habit.

ALCOHOL Excessive drinking can raise blood pressure and the level of damaging fats in the blood, creating a coronary risk. However, moderate drinking of one to two drinks a day generally does not promote heart disease.

HIGH BLOOD PRESSURE Blood pressure readings consistently above 140/90 can indicate a higher than average risk of heart disease. Moderate exercise and relaxation techniques can help to lower blood pressure.

DIABETES The large-scale, long-term Framingham study, involving more than 10,000 people, found that diabetic women had three times higher a risk of coronary artery disease than nondiabetic women. Non-insulin-dependent diabetes mellitus, which is the type of diabetes most common in older people, often involves risk factors of being overweight and having a sedentary lifestyle. If diabetic women maintain healthy blood pressure, cholesterol levels, and weight, their risk of coronary heart disease often decreases.

FAMILY HISTORY Women with parents who suffered a fatal heart attack, particularly if that parent was younger than fifty-five, have an increased risk. This factor often involves cultural eating patterns in addition to genetic factors.

STRESS AND PERSONALITY TYPE The Framingham study found increased coronary artery disease risk in women with certain types of personal, social, and environmental stress. However, since most studies on the Type A personality and stress factors in heart disease have focused on men, the exact role of stress in women's risk is unclear. It is known, however, that people who exercise regularly are better able to withstand the physical effects of stress.

THE POWER OF EXERCISE TO PREVENT HEART DISEASE

▸ ▸ ▸ ▸ ▸ ▸ ▸ ▸ ▸ ▸ ▸

Exercise, along with dietary changes, is instrumental in helping women prevent atherosclerosis and heart disease. From pioneering heart experts such as Dr. Julian Whitaker and Dr. Dean Ornish to cardiologists across the country, doctors are encouraging their patients to exercise regularly and adopt a diet low in animal fat.

Regular exercise conditions the heart to utilize oxygen more efficiently, thereby increasing VO_2max (maximum oxygen consumption). Research has indicated that diminishing VO_2max is not a result of menopause; it is generally due to inactivity, weight gain, and aging. Exercise counteracts two of these factors, enabling postmenopausal women to increase their VO_2max to a healthy level. Studies have shown that moderate aerobic exercise three times a week for twelve weeks can result in a significant increase in VO_2max.

When the heart is conditioned by exercise, it's able to pump more oxygen-rich blood in each beat, resulting in a slower resting pulse rate. The heart has to work less as it works more efficiently.

Exercise has a positive effect on the arteries and can enlarge the arteries to the heart and increase arterial compliance. Exercise also stimulates a protective mechanism which dissolves abnormal blood clots that can block the arteries.

EXERCISE AND CHOLESTEROL

▸ ▸ ▸ ▸ ▸ ▸ ▸ ▸ ▸ ▸ ▸

In addition to conditioning the heart, regular exercise has an impact on cholesterol level. But exercise alone does not significantly lower the level of blood cholesterol. For stronger results, you need to convert to a diet that's low in animal fat.

Some studies have indicated that postmenopausal women who participate in regular endurance exercise have higher HDL cholesterol levels than inactive women. This may be due to the additional positive effects of exercise, such as lower body fat and overall healthy lifestyle. The effect is generally seen after three months of moderate activity. The best results on blood cholesterol are seen when women combine exercise with dietary changes.

BUILDING YOUR AEROBIC POWER

▸ ▸ ▸ ▸ ▸ ▸ ▸ ▸ ▸ ▸ ▸

The most effective type of exercise for preventing heart disease is aerobic exercise (also called cardiorespiratory exercise). In Chapter 8 you'll be introduced to an extensive menu of aerobic choices and guided to select the forms that are appropriate and fun for you.

The classic American College of Sports Medicine (ACSM) guideline for achieving a cardioprotective effect through exercise is: *twenty to sixty minutes of aerobic activity three to five days per week*. This activity should be performed in your Target Heart Rate (THR) zone, which you'll learn to calculate in Chapter 6. Expending 300 calories a day above normal activity range is also a barometer for cardioprotective effect.

If you're not ready to commit to this amount of aerobic exercise, here's some good news: Current thinking in fitness circles is that it's also beneficial to engage in thirty minutes of *cumulative* exercise. In other words, you might do ten minutes on the stationary bike, walk ten minutes to the store, and dance around the kitchen for ten minutes to "bank" your thirty minutes.

In 1995 a panel of twenty experts convened by the Federal Centers for Disease Control and Prevention and the ACSM noted that despite public acceptance of the importance of physical activity for health, the majority of American adults remains essentially sedentary. This inactivity was cited as being responsible for approximately 250,000 deaths per year, or 12 percent of all deaths in the U.S.

The panel encouraged people to incorporate thirty minutes of activity into their daily routines, stating, "Intermittent activity confers substantial benefits." They noted that moderate activity pursued for intervals throughout the day can offer substantial health benefits.

This recommendation has been confirmed in large, long-term studies conducted by leading researcher Dr. Ralph Paffenbarger, at the University of California at Berkeley. Dr. Paffenbarger found that midlife women and men who increased their activity level reduced their chances of all causes of morbidity and mortality.

To put it plainly: *It's never too late or too little.*

During the 4-Week Workout Program you're encouraged to exercise aerobically for at least twenty minutes at least three times a week. Hopefully, you'll find you enjoy this routine enough to continue it indefinitely. But if you simply can't find the time or discipline for a regimented program, you have a choice: You can take ten minutes here and there throughout the day to bank your physical activity. It's a worthwhile investment for a healthy heart and future.

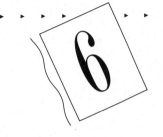

6

FINDING YOUR
FITNESS LEVEL

Every midlife woman has the capacity to enjoy a safe exercise program and work her way to fitness. Whether you've been exercising regularly, occasionally, or rarely, the 4-Week Workout Program can be adapted to your individual condition and needs. The key is to consult with your health professional first, and then identify your personal fitness level.

Before beginning this program or starting any new exercise, it is essential that you have a complete physical examination and get your physician's go-ahead.

Even if you already exercise regularly and feel in great shape, you need to have a medical examination. Only a qualified doctor can determine whether or not you have any hidden conditions of which you may not be aware.

If you have any medical conditions, injuries, disabilities, orthopedic or bone concerns, you should consult with your health professional to determine how you can adapt the exercise recommendations in this book. Then you can participate in new exercise activities with peace of mind.

WARNING SIGNS

The exercise philosophy of "no pain, no gain" is outmoded and dangerous. While you may experience some discomfort or strain during exercise, you should never be in agony.

If you experience the following warning signs during or after exercise, *stop working out* and go for a thorough medical examination as soon as possible. Be aware that these are only *some* of the possible warning signs:

- Extremely rapid or irregular heartbeat
- Shortness of breath or difficulty breathing
- Dizziness or fainting
- Sudden, sharp, or recurrent pain

Listen to your body while you exercise and respect the messages it sends. There's a subtle line between a healthy challenge and pushing yourself too far. It's always better to be a little cautious, especially if you're not at a top fitness level. You want to stay well so you can continue to exercise on a regular basis, since it's regularity that counts in the long run.

"Weekend warriors" who suddenly throw themselves into intense physical activity are more likely to be injured. Be sensible and protect yourself.

YOUR PERSONAL FITNESS LEVEL

Identifying your personal fitness level will help you select appropriate forms of aerobic exercise and determine the intensity and duration of the sessions. This will also guide you through the strength-training workouts, which have variations for different fitness levels.

The personal fitness levels are a tool, not a judgment. These levels will guide you to an exercise program that is not too difficult and overwhelming. Be honest and careful in selecting your level and don't worry if you begin in level 1. After a few months of regular exercise, you're likely to find yourself moving up a level. The primary goal is to start and stay with a balanced exercise program and to progress gradually.

The fitness levels for this program are determined by these basic criteria:

- Number of coronary risk factors
- Aerobic test
- Strength test
- Experience
- Any injuries, illnesses, or conditions you may have

CORONARY RISK FACTORS

One of the elements of your fitness level is the number of coronary risk factors you may have in your medical profile. The American College of Sports Medicine has developed the following criteria for assessing your coronary risk factors:

1. Diagnosed hypertension blood pressure ≥ 140/90 mm Hg on at least two separate occasions, or on antihypertensive medication
2. Total serum cholesterol > 200 mg/dL or HDL < 35 mg/dL
3. Cigarette smoking
4. Diabetes mellitus
5. Family history of coronary or other atherosclerotic disease in parents or siblings prior to age fifty-five.

Major symptoms or signs suggestive of cardiopulmonary or metabolic disease include:

1. Pain or discomfort in the chest or surrounding areas that appears to be ischemic in nature.
2. Unaccustomed shortness of breath or shortness of breath with mild exertion.
3. Dizziness
4. Orthopnea/paroxysmal nocturnal dyspnea (nighttime labored breathing)
5. Ankle edema
6. Palpitations or tachycardia
7. Claudication (aching, weakness, or cramping, usually in the calf) during physical activity
8. Known heart murmur

NOTE: If you have two or more of the coronary risk factors, and/or one or more signs or symptoms, consult with your physician before beginning *any* exercise program. A consultation should include a medical examination and clinical exercise test.

THE AEROBIC AND STRENGTH TESTS

Other criteria for determining your fitness level involve two simple tests: a walk or run test to measure aerobic fitness, and modified pushups to measure strength.

You may find you're at a certain level for aerobic ability and at a different level for strength. This indicates that you should use the appropriate level when choosing the type, duration, and intensity of your aerobic workout, and the other level when doing the 4-Week Workouts for strength training.

AEROBIC TEST Time how long it takes you to walk or run 1.5 miles. If you're not an experienced runner, stick to walking for this test. You can measure your time on a treadmill with a digital read-out, or on a 1.5-mile walking course. You can measure outdoor distance by driving down the street and reading your odometer before walking the same route, or by using a pedometer, which you can purchase in a sporting goods store.

STRENGTH TEST See how many modified pushups you can do without feeling great strain. To do modified pushups, go onto your hands and knees, cross your ankles, and lift your feet off the floor. Lower yourself down and lift yourself up slowly, being careful not to arch your back. Make a note of how many pushups you can do comfortably.

After you have completed these physical tests and noted the results, you are ready to determine your fitness level according to the following criteria. If you ran during the aerobic test, decrease the time limit specified in the fitness levels by seven minutes.

LEVEL 1
Two or more major coronary risk factors.
New to exercise.
Consider yourself at below average fitness level.
Recovering from an injury, working with modifications.
Time for 1.5-mile walk/run is over twenty-seven minutes.
Can comfortably do less than seven modified pushups.

LEVEL 2
One or no major coronary risk factors.
Familiar with and have participated in exercise or sports.
May have chronic joint and muscle discomfort but familiar with
    limitations.
Consider yourself at an average fitness level.
Can walk/run 1.5 miles in twenty-four to twenty-seven minutes.
Can do seven to fourteen modified pushups.

LEVEL 3
One or no major coronary risk factors.
Have been participating regularly in a fitness program.
Consider yourself at a high fitness level.
Can walk/run 1.5 miles in under twenty-four minutes.
Can do more than fifteen modified pushups.

FOR WOMEN WITH OSTEOPOROSIS If you have been diagnosed with osteoporosis, you should not choose a fitness level according to the above criteria. Instead, please refer to the aerobic and special workout recommendations in Chapter 17.

YOUR RPE

▸ ▸ ▸ ▸ ▸ ▸ ▸ ▸ ▸ ▸

Once you start exercising it can be helpful to use two methods to measure the intensity of your aerobic sessions: the Rated Perceived Exertion (RPE) and the Target Heart Rate (THR) zone.

The Borg Scale of RPE is a simple means of determining the

intensity of aerobic exercise. Since this measurement is subjective, it is not always as accurate as monitoring the heart rate, but it can be easier to do. The RPE can help you maintain a comfortable yet challenging level of intensity.

The RPE is measured by how hard you *perceive* you are working during aerobic exercise, according to this scale:

6	
7	VERY, VERY LIGHT
8	
9	VERY LIGHT
10	
11	FAIRLY LIGHT
12	
13	SOMEWHAT HARD
14	
15	HARD
16	
17	VERY HARD
18	
19	VERY, VERY HARD
20	

Borg, G.A.V., "Psychological Bases of Physical Exertion," *Medicine and Science in Sport and Exercise*, ACSM 14 (1982): 377–87. Reprinted with permission.

If you are in fitness level 1, your aerobic activity should be performed in the 11–13 range. If you are in fitness level 2, work in the 13–15 RPE range. And if you are in fitness level 3, your RPE during aerobic activity should be in the 13–17 zone.

HOW TO DETERMINE YOUR TARGET HEART RATE ZONE

▸ ▸ ▸ ▸ ▸ ▸ ▸ ▸ ▸ ▸

The THR zone is a tool for measuring the cardiorespiratory benefits of your aerobic workout. It helps you work at an intensity that's safe for your heart and maximally beneficial.

The following formula for determining your THR zone may seem complicated, but if you use a pencil, pad, and calculator, it's a cinch.

Once you know your THR zone, you don't need to do the arithmetic again. All you need to do is measure your pulse about ten minutes into your aerobic workouts and see if you're in your zone. If you're not, you need to accelerate the intensity or slow it down to achieve the THR zone.

To determine your THR zone:

1. Using your first two fingers, find your pulse on the thumb side of your wrist (with palm up) or in the groove of your neck (carotid artery).

Using a watch or clock with a secon[d]
of beats in ten seconds, then multiply b[y]
heart rate (RHR). To get an accurate re[a]
secutive mornings when you first wake [up in]
bed. Make a note of your RHR.

A normal resting heart rate is 60–80 b[eats]

2. Use a piece of scratch paper to make the
to determine your THR using the Karvo[nen]
example given is for a fifty-year-old woman with a resting heart
rate of 72. The starting figure of 220 is standard for everyone.

Subtract your age	220
	−50
Your maximum heart rate	170
Subtract your resting heart rate	−72
Your heart rate reserve	98
Multiply by 60%	×.60
	58.8
Add RHR	+72
	130.8
Your heart rate reserve multiplied by 80%	98
	×.80
	78.4
Add RHR	+72
	150.4
Round off the two figures:	131–150

For the woman in this example, the THR for aerobic exercise is
131–150 beats per minute, which is 60 to 80 percent of her maximum heart rate.

BODY MASS INDEX
▸ ▸ ▸ ▸ ▸ ▸ ▸ ▸ ▸ ▸ ▸

Although many women are concerned about their weight on the
scale, this is a misguided preoccupation since pounds are not an
accurate indication of fitness or of whether you look fat. There are
too many other variables.

A muscular woman in excellent shape can weigh more than a
flabby woman with little muscle. A woman with a lot of curves
may weigh more than a less well-endowed woman yet appear to be
thinner. There is, in reality, no such thing as the perfect weight for
a certain height. Nonetheless, many women are determined to
know whether they are "overweight" or at a healthy weight.

If you are interested in fat assessment, a more accurate measurement than the bathroom scale is the Body Mass Index (BMI), which is your weight over your height squared (weight/height^2).

You can calculate your BMI on the chart below by placing a dot to indicate how many pounds you usually weigh in the middle of the day. Then place a dot to mark your height. Using a ruler or straightedge, connect the dots. Note the number on the middle scale where your line intersects it. This number indicates your BMI.

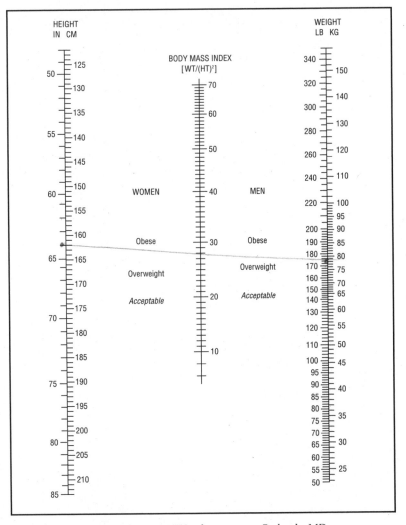

Bray, G.A., ed. *Obesity in America*. NIH pub. no. 79-359. Bethesda, MD.

According to William Evans, Ph.D.,author of *Biomarkers* and director of the Noll Physiological Research Center at Penn State University, these are the ideal BMIs for midlife women:

Age 40–49   23.2
Age 50–59   25.2

If your BMI is 20 percent or more above these ideal figures, this indicates a weight problem that can increase your risk of developing a chronic disease and dying prematurely. A BMI of 28 or over is considered overweight and increases the likelihood of health problems.

The BMI should be considered a tool for assessment rather than a definitive marker of fitness. Be aware that the BMI has a flaw: It does not precisely measure body fat and anatomical position of fat (for example, waist-to-hip ratio).

BODY FAT PERCENTAGE (BFP)

▶ ▶ ▶ ▶ ▶ ▶ ▶ ▶ ▶ ▶ ▶

If you'd like to go a step further and measure your body fat percentage, you'll need the assistance of a health professional who can do the testing and assess the results. There are several methods:

SKIN FOLD MEASUREMENT This can be done with calipers by a doctor or an exercise physiologist. It is one of the most accessible ways to measure BFP.

ELECTRODE METHOD This measurement technique is performed in a clinical setting (doctor's office, hospital, or clinic) using bioelectrical impedance analysis.

DENSITOMETRY–DEXA This stands for dual energy x-ray absorptiometry, an FDA approved evaluation of body composition and bone density now available to the public.

HYDROSTATIC WEIGHING Since this technique involves submersion under water, it can only be performed in a special clinical or lab setting. It is known as the gold standard of body fat testing for its accuracy.

The distribution of your body fat, as well as the percentage, is a factor in fitness and longevity. There is evidence that people who store the majority of their fat around the waist rather than around the hips or thighs run the greatest risk of developing heart disease, stroke, and Type II diabetes.

If you have extra body fat, it's better to be shaped like a pear than an apple. The waist-to-hip ratio is the circumference of the waist divided by the circumference of the hips. Ratios of .86 or above increase health risks.

Whatever your BMI, BFP, or fat distribution, many studies have shown that exercise, along with a sensible diet, is the best way to lose body fat as you maintain or gain muscle.

7

THE ELEMENTS

OF EXERCISE

Midlife women, like all people who want to be fit and healthy, need a balanced exercise program that includes the three components of exercise:

> "Exercise is crucial for midlife women. All forms of exercise are beneficial. Yoga and stretching are excellent for maintaining flexibility, and aerobic exercise is excellent for maintaining heart and lung health. Bones need all of the above, but also exercise where strengthening is involved."
>
> —RICHARD BOCKMAN, M.D., PH.D.
>
> Professor of Medicine, Cornell University Medical Center

▸ Aerobic activity (cardiorespiratory endurance)
▸ Strength training (muscle strength)
▸ Flexibility exercise (stretching)

A well-rounded exercise program is like a balanced diet: you need a certain amount of each type of nourishment each week for optimum health. In the following chapters, you'll learn how to select from an enticing and varied menu of exercise choices. Here's an introduction to the basic elements.

AEROBIC ACTIVITY

Aerobic or cardiorespiratory exercise is any activity that uses the large muscles in a sustained motion over a period of time. Aerobic activity is measured by intensity and duration.

The ACSM publishes a position paper on "The Recommended Quantity and Quality of Exercise for Developing and Maintaining Cardiorespiratory and Muscular Fitness in Healthy Adults." This provides the basic guidelines for personal trainers and fitness practitioners.

The ACSM recommends the following aerobic exercise prescription:

FREQUENCY: three to five aerobic training sessions per week

INTENSITY: 60 to 90 percent of maximum heart rate (HRmax), or 50 to 85 percent of maximum oxygen uptake (VO$_2$max)

DURATION: twenty to sixty minutes of continuous aerobic activity

As part of the 4-Week Workout Program, you'll be doing at least three aerobic activities a week. User-friendly charts will help you determine the appropriate duration for your particular fitness level and activity. Whenever working aerobically, it's recommended to stay in your THR zone.

Some women are intimidated by the term "aerobics" and picture superfit women in thong leotards jumping up and down with boundless energy. You may be encouraged to know that, if done with sufficient intensity and duration, walking and swimming can qualify as aerobic.

Other aerobic activities include hiking, running, jogging, bicycling, aerobic dancing, step classes, and stair climbing. And for added variety there's cross-country skiing, skating, and team sports.

In addition to reducing the risk of heart disease and osteoporosis, aerobic exercise also helps you do the following:

▸ Decrease the risk of Type II (adult onset) diabetes by helping to maintain normal glucose and triglyceride levels.
▸ Increase the body's ability to utilize oxygen.
▸ Fight the physical effects of stress and survive a cardiac event.
▸ Increase metabolic rate and maintain a desirable body weight.

Will aerobic activity enable you to shed any or all of the extra weight you may want to lose? The answer depends on your diet and your genetic makeup as well as your exercise program. However, this much is certain: Aerobic activity done at a low to moderate intensity for a sufficient duration uses both glucose (carbohydrates) and free fatty acids for fuel. Physical activity has a profound effect on increasing metabolism.

Whether you want to lose weight, maintain your figure after menopause, or turn body fat into lean muscle mass, aerobic activity is essential. And the longer you work out, the more calories you use.

STRENGTH TRAINING

▸ ▸ ▸ ▸ ▸ ▸ ▸ ▸ ▸ ▸ ▸

Strength training, also known as muscle strength exercises, works individual muscle groups to increase strength. It involves building muscle power while working against resistance created by free weights, mechanical weights, or body weight.

In 1990 the ACSM revised their exercise guidelines to recommend a more balanced fitness program that includes strength training along with aerobic activity. It is now recommended that people do at least two strength workouts a week, consisting of at least one set of eight to twelve repetitions (reps) of eight to ten exercises that condition the major muscle groups.

If these numbers make your head spin, don't worry. The Strength Training Routine provides sufficient sets and reps in an easy-to-follow sequence. You'll move through the routines to your favorite music and fifteen to twenty minutes later you'll have worked all your major muscle groups.

Other strength-training activities include lifting free weights using resistance machines such as Nautilus, or using exercise bands. You can also use your own body weight as resistance when doing pushups, sit-ups, and other calisthenics.

The Strength Training Routines are designed to give you gain without pain and strengthen all the major muscle groups in a manageable way. You'll probably enjoy the workouts, and you'll definitely appreciate the benefits.

In addition to its influence on bone health and osteoporosis, strength training gives you the stability to reduce your risk of falling, fractures, and other injuries. It also has a dramatic impact on your body composition. *Strength training helps you lose fat and build muscle.* It increases metabolic rate so you use more calories and maintain fat-free weight. And it leads to a greater sense of physical and emotional power.

FLEXIBILITY

▸ ▸ ▸ ▸ ▸ ▸ ▸ ▸ ▸ ▸ ▸

Stretching, or flexibility exercise, is the third element of a comprehensive workout regime. Stretching offers these benefits:

- ▸ Increased range of motion and flexibility
- ▸ Decreased risk of injury and muscle soreness
- ▸ Reduced risk of back and neck pain from everyday stresses
- ▸ Enhanced body alignment and posture
- ▸ Alleviation of the physical and emotional effects of stress

If you've ever watched a cat or a dog, you know that stretching is a natural instinct. Cats move into a series of stretches throughout the day, and dogs stretch forward in a "play bow" to signal they're ready to frolic. For us humans, stretching is a pleasurable treat for bodies that are crammed into chairs, clothes, and other unnatural constrictions for much of the day.

Stretching is done both as a warm-up and a cooldown for aerobic and strength workouts. As part of the program, you'll be doing Warm-up and Flexibility Cooldown routines before and after workouts. This means you'll be doing a stretching sequence at least five times a week. My recommendation is that you do a few stretches *every day* to invigorate and relax.

ENJOY YOUR EXERCISE
▸ ▸ ▸ ▸ ▸ ▸ ▸ ▸ ▸ ▸ ▸

Alice, a forty-four-year-old graphic artist, has an extremely busy freelance career and often works into the night. Yet no matter what deadlines loom, she always goes to the gym for aerobic step and strength classes. She finds the time because she loves the workouts and the rewards.

"I don't care how busy I am, the gym is my time for myself and I fit it in somehow. The classes are so much fun and they let me completely forget about all the pressure. I just lose myself in the music and the concentration and challenge. And afterwards, instead of being tired, I have more energy to do what I need to do. I can concentrate on work because I've had my fun."

Do you wonder what separates people who exercise regularly from fitness dropouts? The people who stay with it are generally those who *enjoy* exercise. It's not a big surprise. If you're forcing yourself to do something because you think you *should*, it won't be long before you rebel. But if you choose forms of fitness that are fun, you'll be more inclined to keep going.

You may be worried about osteoporosis, heart disease, and aging and know that you need to exercise. Still, unless you find a workout that's pleasurable, the fear may not be enough motivation to keep you going.

According to a 1994 *New York Times* article, even after decades of health experts urging Americans to exercise, only 20 percent of the population does the minimum required for fitness (fifteen to twenty minutes of moderate exercise three times a week). Another poll, sponsored by the President's Council on Physical Fitness and Sports in 1993, found that 41 percent of the U.S. adult population "failed to engage in vigorous exercise even two times a week."

It's clear that the threat of disease and obesity alone are not enough to get people moving. That's why I promote the pleasure principle of exercise. Positive conditioning is much more successful than fear. The best way to avoid being an exercise dropout is to follow your pleasure. Experiment and explore until you find the form of exercise that delights you.

VARIETY IS THE SPICE

▶ ▶ ▶ ▶ ▶ ▶ ▶ ▶ ▶ ▶ ▶

With all the myriad of physical activities to explore, there's no reason ever to be bored with exercise. If you find exercise dull, it may be time to find a more challenging activity.

One of the qualities of youth that people miss most is the excitement of new experiences. The world of fitness is a wonderful place to renew your adventurous spirit.

Although it can be a little scary to try new activities, this type of fear is a healthy antidote to the daily grind of stress we face. Physical adventures can take you soaring above your daily concerns and leave you feeling renewed and powerful.

You don't need to hike up a remote mountain or ski down a slope to savor the thrill of new physical experiences. You might choose to take up racquetball or start ballet classes instead. Whatever you try that's different and challenging will give you a lift. Even if you think of yourself as a nonathletic person, you can discover ways to be more active than ever before.

One reason some women get depressed when they go through menopause is because it represents diminishing possibilities. Women may feel that after menopause "There are so many things I'll never do, now that I'm no longer young."

Exercise is a powerful way to counteract this negative mindset. It can help you break out of your routine and experience your powerful potential. You can take a jazz dance class and feel like a Broadway star; take a brisk walk and lose yourself in the beauty of nature; go for a bike ride and feel like a kid again. The activities you can do to lift yourself out of the ordinary are unlimited.

Remember when you were a little girl and you couldn't wait to go outside and play? Or you eagerly participated in an after-school sport or dance class? Exercise can bring that sense of playfulness and fun back into your life. You can enjoy the confidence and know-how of midlife along with the sheer exuberance of youth.

8

CHOOSING THE AEROBIC ACTIVITY THAT'S RIGHT FOR YOU

Aerobic exercise is important for both men and women, at all ages, to reduce the risk of heart disease and enhance overall health. What's different for midlife women is the need to select a form of aerobic activity that has great impact on bone health as well as on the cardiorespiratory system: a weight-bearing exercise.

Weight-bearing aerobic exercise is any activity done standing. This includes:

- Walking and hiking (outside or on a treadmill)
- Running/jogging (outside or on a treadmill)
- Stepping (on a step platform, in a class, or following a video)
- Stair climbing (on a stair machine or on stairs)
- Dancing (aerobic dance classes, some forms of jazz and social dancing)
- Cross-country skiing (outside or on a ski machine)

Non-weight-bearing aerobic activities are ones that are not done standing. These include:

- Swimming
- Biking (outside or on a stationary bike)
- Rowing (outside or on a rowing machine)

The National Osteoporosis Foundation states: "Weight-bearing exercise, such as walking, hiking, stair climbing, or jogging is recommended over non-weight-bearing exercise such as swimming or cycling, although some type of physical activity is better than nothing."

This statement reinforces one of the principles of my own exercise philosophy: *Something is better than nothing.*

While there are always ideals in an exercise program, the primary goal is to get up and do something active on a regular basis.

If you love to swim or cycle, don't stop! Just add one or two sessions of brisk walking each week, and two sessions of strength-training exercises to keep your bones strong. Remember the pleasure principle and continue any exercise you enjoy.

WALKING AND HIKING

Walking is probably the most popular and universal form of exercise throughout the world. It's cost-free and natural; in fact, if we walked the way nature intended, we might not need exercise programs at all.

You should be aware, however, that a sunset stroll or a walk to the corner store is not necessarily aerobic, although it's better than sitting. Whether or not a walk is aerobic depends on its intensity and duration.

To gain cardiorespiratory benefits, you need to walk at an intensity where you feel that your heart is pumping and your breath is faster than it is while you're resting. You need to walk up and down hills or move briskly on a flat surface.

A brisk thirty-minute walk that includes some hills will meet your requirements. If you live in a flat area, accelerate your speed once you've warmed up and walk quickly for at least fifteen minutes out of thirty.

Walking up and down hills increases the aerobic effect. It's not necessary to walk faster up the hill; the slope itself will increase your heart rate. If there's just one hill on your walking route, go up and down it several times to maximize the challenge. Take it slowly when you're walking down hills since this puts pressure on your joints.

Be sure you have good walking sneakers, sports socks, and comfortable clothes with pockets for your keys. Start by walking slowly for the first five minutes to warm up. Then gradually accelerate your pace. Slow down again for the last five minutes of your walk.

I do not recommend using hand-held weights or ankle weights

while walking. The extra weight puts stress on your joints and can cause more injury than good.

After walking, and all aerobic activities, it's important to do the Flexibility Cooldown routine that follows the Strength Training Routine, or to do other gentle stretches.

Many women enjoy walking with friends, both for the companionship and to be sure they get out there and do it. Children and dogs also make terrific walking partners. On the other hand, you may also enjoy walking alone and using it as a quiet, contemplative, creative time.

Although treadmill walking may not be as pleasant as being outdoors, it does have its advantages. It will get you moving on days when it's rainy or cold outside. If you're bored by outdoor walks, you can watch TV or listen to music on the treadmill. High-tech treadmills give you digital information about your walking speed and distance, heart rate, and calorie expenditure.

Hiking or taking lengthy outdoor walks is a rugged experience that involves a bigger time commitment than the thirty-minute fitness walk. Hiking is a great escape, if you're well prepared and have no injuries or serious medical conditions. You can condition yourself for hiking by walking for at least one hour three times a week for three months (being sure to include uphill terrain). Whenever you go hiking in the wilderness, bring a companion and plenty of water.

Walking is recommended for all fitness levels. See the chart at the end of this chapter for appropriate intensity and duration. Hiking is appropriate for Fitness Level 3, and for Fitness Level 2 with training.

JOGGING/RUNNING

One of the most exciting events of my life was running 26.2 miles in the New York City Marathon only six months after a serious bicycle accident and nine years after an intense dance-related knee injury. The thrill came from meeting a goal that sometimes seemed impossible, and achieving that goal along with 26,000 other lunatics.

At the twenty-four-mile mark of the marathon one of my clients, Carol, joined me for a half-mile run. Carol (who is one of our models for this book) was forty-nine years old at the time and had started a regular aerobic exercise program only a year before.

We had started Carol's conditioning with brisk walks around the Central Park Reservoir, then added short bursts of jogging. Sometimes we'd jog to catch up with a star we spotted running in the park—Madonna, Robert Redford, or Harrison Ford. After a few months we achieved Carol's goal of running around the entire reservoir, a 1.6-mile course. But we never achieved my goal of running into John Kennedy Jr. on the path.

Carol had neither the time nor the desire to train to run the full New York City Marathon, but we both thought it would be fun if she ran part of the course. Seeing the proud look on her face as we ran side by side gave me a burst of energy that I desperately needed after twenty-four miles.

Although running is an arduous activity, it's not exclusively for young people. Many midlife women who take up running feel that no other fitness activity matches it for the sheer sense of exhilaration and accomplishment, as well as the heart benefits.

Yet despite all its pluses, running also has its downside. It's a high-impact activity and puts a lot of stress on the bones, joints, and heart. Running is recommended only for midlife women who are basically healthy and do not have arthritis, low bone density or osteoporosis, a heart condition, injuries, or orthopedic concerns. *Before you start a running program, it's essential to have a complete physical examination.*

If your doctor gives you the go-ahead, first you need to qualify as a strong walker before you start running. You should be able to walk three times a week for thirty minutes in your THR zone without straining. After you have done this for two weeks, you can add one minute of slow jogging to every five minutes of walking. Approach this activity in a methodical manner: Be a strong walker before you jog and a strong jogger before you run.

Once you're off and running you can gradually build up your frequency, duration, and intensity. For midlife women, it's best to focus on increasing duration and frequency instead of intensity or speed. There's not enough difference in the bone benefits to risk the injury involved in high-speed running.

Check your heart rate when you're about ten minutes into the run to be sure you're in the target zone. You can do this with the method given in Chapter 6, or with a heart rate monitoring device you can buy at a sporting goods store. If your heart rate is too high, slow down your pace.

Another guideline to remember is that you should be able to talk, but not sing, during aerobic activity. It's fun to run with a friend and chat—or talk about how hard it is! Running is not a stroll through the daisies, and a little complaining is good for the soul.

Jogging or running requires comfortable, quality gear: running sneakers built for the forward motion; sport socks to absorb water away from the skin; light, layered clothing appropriate for the season; and a supportive sports bra. You'll need a pocket or pouch for your keys and reflective patches if you're running in the evening.

Jogging or running on a treadmill is a handy option for rainy or cold weather (or if you feel unsafe running in your neighborhood). Machines come in a wide range of styles, from simple treadmills to high-tech models that tell you everything but your horoscope. The high-tech models offer a variety of speed and "terrain," and are useful if you don't get too focused on the digital readouts. Get into your own rhythm and enjoy.

To warm up for jogging or running, do some mild stretching, then run slowly for the first five minutes. To cool down, walk for the last five minutes of the session, then do a stretching session when you're finished.

Even if you feel like flopping on the sofa after a run, you need to resist the impulse and force yourself to stretch to reduce the risk of soreness and injury. It's also nice to take a strong, hot shower or a leisurely bath to relax those hard-working muscles and joints.

Jogging and running are appropriate for Fitness Level 3, and for Fitness Level 2 with training.

STEPPING

▶ ▶

In the old days, people bitterly complained about living in walk-up buildings with no elevators. Now they're hopping up and down steps of their own free will.

Stepping is a relatively new activity created as a low-impact workout. It caught on like wildfire, and step classes and videos are now extremely popular.

Stepping is an excellent weight-bearing aerobic activity for midlife women, with strong cardiovascular and bone benefits. It allows you to work in your THR zone without great strain and strengthens bone with low impact. You can step at home or with a group in a class. Step classes incorporate the challenge of choreography and dance with a thorough workout.

Stepping is energizing and allows you to gain big benefits in a small space. It's a relatively safe activity, although not for all women with orthopedic concerns or injuries.

Sneakers designed for step classes, aerobic dance, or cross training are fine for step sessions. Many women like to wear snazzy dance-style leotards. Let your outfit reflect your personality and style.

If you want to do your stepping at home, you need to purchase a step, which is essentially a platform on blocks. They come in various sizes, and your height and experience will determine the height of your step. Ask an exercise instructor or knowledgeable sporting goods salesperson for guidance.

Step classes are now offered at health clubs, gyms, dance studios, YWCAs or YMCAs, and continuing education centers. When choosing a class, it's a good idea to start with a basic one so you aren't confused by the choreography. The class should have appropriate step-tempo music (about 120 beats per minute) and a teacher in whom you have confidence. If you have trouble following along, focus on doing the leg movements, then add the arms when you're comfortable with the steps.

You can also follow a step class on a variety of videos. Try renting a tape at the video store to see if it's the right one for you before making a purchase. Even if you are at a high fitness level, start with a beginner step video until you get accustomed to the choreography and the coordination of the movements.

Your knees should always be slightly bent while stepping, your shoulders aligned with your hips, and your back straight. Keep an eye on the step and place your whole foot on it. If your knees hurt during or after a step session, you may need to lower the height of your step.

Step classes and videotapes generally take a half-hour to an hour, and include warm-up, cooldown, and stretching portions. You may want to do additional gentle stretching afterwards.

Stair machines, which preceded the more lovable step, can be a vigorous aerobic and weight-bearing workout. Some women who want a no-nonsense workout to firm up their legs and buttocks swear by the stair machines, which are usually found in health clubs.

Stepping and stairs are recommended for all fitness levels. Women with osteoporosis should consult their doctor to see if it is suitable.

AEROBIC DANCING, DANCE CLASSES, AND SOCIAL DANCING

The fitness revolution was ignited by the craze for high-impact aerobic dance classes. Then many women were turned off by the overly energetic routines and high rate of injury. The good news is that these problems spurred fitness professionals to find a way to gain the same benefits without the injuries, and the low-impact aerobic dance class was born.

Low-impact means at least one foot stays on the floor at all times and there are no jarring jumping movements. Almost all aerobic dance classes are low-impact these days, and for midlife women it's the preferred way to go.

Low-impact aerobic dancing is a weight-bearing activity with solid cardiorespiratory and bone benefits. It helps coordination and posture and lets you feel like a dancer. If you enjoy moving to music, aerobic dancing is a delightful way to work out. All you need to start are sneakers that are designed for this activity and comfortable workout clothes.

Aerobic dance classes are offered in gyms, health clubs, YWCAs or YMCAs, dance studios, and continuing education centers. Inquire into the fitness credentials of the instructor to be sure she or he is qualified and experienced. It's helpful if you can watch a class or get a recommendation from someone who has worked with the instructor before signing up.

The quality of an aerobic dance class depends to a large degree on the instructor, and styles vary widely. The teacher should be encouraging but not intimidating, and should watch the students for form and technique. If you're trying aerobic dance for the first time or resuming after a long hiatus, take a beginner class.

If you enjoy aerobic dance, you can experiment with different styles. In some areas you can find classes with themes: line dancing, Afro-Caribbean, jazz, or rock-and-roll aerobic dance.

There's also a wide assortment of aerobic dance videos you can use at home. If possible, rent from the video store before purchasing a tape to make sure it's worthwhile.

In addition to aerobics, you might try other types of dance classes: jazz, ballet, modern, belly dancing. These are generally anaerobic, which means they involve stop-and-start movements. Depending on the class, dance has varying degrees of cardiorespiratory effects, and can also benefit your bones, muscles, and flexibility. Best of all, dance classes get you moving to the music.

If you've always wanted to wear a sequined bra and harem pants, take a Middle Eastern dance class. If you want to go back to the ballet classes you gave up when you were twelve, try it out. It's terrific to explore new personas in midlife and realize you never stop learning and changing.

Another weight-bearing aerobic/anaerobic activity is social dancing, which can be ballroom, disco, rock, country and western, square dancing, or line dancing. These forms of dance can provide a solid workout if you move continuously for twenty minutes or longer. The music and your partners can inspire you to keep moving.

Low-impact aerobic dance, dance classes, and social dancing are recommended for all fitness levels. Women with osteoporosis should check with their doctor before participating in these activities.

SKIING AND SKATING

If you're adventurous, you may want to try other weight-bearing aerobic activities such as cross-country skiing, ice skating, or in-line skating. For these sports you need quality skis or skates, protective gear, and lessons. The risk of injury can be high, and a mature woman shouldn't hurl herself across the snow, ice, or pavement without preparation. Also, if you have low bone density or osteoporosis, avoid these activities since they put you at higher risk for falls and fractures.

Although opportunities to ski across outdoor trails are limited, many health clubs offer machines to simulate the movement. If you prefer, you can purchase a ski machine for your home gym.

To gain effective cardiorespiratory benefits, you need to use a ski machine for at least twenty minutes. You also can combine a ten-minute workout on this device with sessions on other aerobic machines in a circuit.

Outdoor cross-country skiing and skating are appropriate for Fitness Level 3, and Fitness Level 2 with experience. Indoor ski machines can be used by Fitness Levels 2 and 3; by Fitness Level 1, with supervision.

RACQUET AND OTHER SPORTS

Like all sports that are played on your feet, tennis and racquetball are weight-bearing activities and have benefits for your bones and muscles. Since the action is not constantly sustained, these sports are a cross between aerobic and anaerobic, involving short bursts of high-intensity activity.

Many midlife women adore racquet sports for the combination of skill, competition, and social activity. There's something about smashing a dynamite serve over the net and watching your partner dive for it that's incredibly satisfying.

If you play a serious game of singles three times a week, this will help to keep your heart and muscles strong. However, you should add a strength workout (such as the Strength Training Routine) twice a week to systematically strengthen your bones and muscles. You may also want to do additional reps of the arm exercises on the side you don't use to swing your racquet, to balance out muscle development.

Golf, like many social sports, is more a game of skill than an aerobic exercise. It has some cardiorespiratory and bone benefits, but only if the course is walked. Although riding around in a golf cart is a delightful way to spend a Sunday, it doesn't do much for the heart. If golf is your game, try to do at least two sessions of aerobic activity a week and two strength workouts. This can also improve your golf game.

More and more, midlife women are participating in a variety of team sports: basketball, soccer, volleyball, even baseball and hockey. These competitive sports are a wonderful way to reduce tension and work up a sweat. However, to achieve balanced fitness, you should supplement sports with systematic aerobic and strength workouts. These workouts will also improve skill, strength, and coordination for your favorite game.

Whatever sport you play, proper warm-up and cooldown are required to reduce the chance of injury.

Tennis, racquetball, golf, and other sports are recommended for Fitness Level 3, and Fitness Level 2 with sufficient preparation and practice. Fitness Level 1 women may be able to play sports with caution and practice. Women with osteoporosis should avoid these activities as they can increase your risk of fractures.

SWIMMING

Swimming is a safe aerobic activity that's excellent for cardiorespiratory and overall fitness. If you swim for twenty minutes or more three times a week, you can feel assured that you're doing well by your heart.

Swimming is also good for strengthening muscles, especially in the upper body, since the water adds resistance to the movement. It's therapeutic for rehabilitating injured joints and for arthritis. The rhythmic nature of swimming and immersion in water makes it soothing for the mind as well as the body.

Although swimming is considered the perfect exercise by many people, it has one major drawback: *Swimming is a non-weight-bearing activity.* Since the water supports your body weight, it doesn't build bone strength and does little to help the problem of low bone density. Also, swimming does a lot more to condition the upper body than the lower.

If you love to swim, remember the pleasure principle and keep on stroking. But you need to add twice-weekly muscle-strength workouts to your fitness routine and, if possible, a session of weight-bearing aerobic activity at least once a week.

The equipment for swimming is obvious: a comfortable bathing suit, goggles, and a swim cap. Follow safety precautions and never swim alone. The injury rate in swimming is low compared to many activities, providing you're sensible.

Some women like to use hand paddles or fins to add resistance to their swimming workout. These gadgets can build strength and endurance, but you need to be careful not to overwork muscles suddenly.

There are many amusing ways to work out in the water besides lap swimming. You can do your warm-up and cooldown stretching right in the pool. You can walk and run in the water or take aqua aerobic classes. And if you're lucky, you can float on a raft when you're done and have someone hand you a cold mint iced tea!

Swimming is appropriate for all fitness levels and for women with osteoporosis.

CYCLING

I enjoy cycling more than any other form of exercise and for years it was my main aerobic activity. I thought I was doing very well since bicycling is a superior cardiorespiratory workout, but once I began studying osteoporosis, I realized that cycling is not a weight-bearing activity. It was necessary to add a weight-bearing workout to my fitness regime.

Bicycling, either outdoors or on a stationary bike, has substantial benefits for the heart if you do it continuously for at least twenty minutes, and it has some benefits for the bone, particularly in the lumbar spine. However, if this is your primary exercise, you need to supplement it with regular strength workouts and weight-bearing aerobic activity.

For outdoor biking there's one piece of equipment that's a matter of life and death: a high-quality helmet. You'll also need sneakers with a good grip and biking shorts or pants. It's advisable to ride with a bike pump, a spare inner tube, a repair kit, a bottle of water, and the number of your local taxi service in case all else fails.

Touring or racing bikes are favored by experienced bikers who want to travel long distances. Hybrid bikes, a combination of touring and mountain bikes, can be easier to handle when you're starting out. The hybrids are ridden in a more upright position, which is easier on the spine and back. They have thicker tires for a greater sense of stability.

Indoor stationary bikes are another alternative, although you miss the glory of watching the world go by. Indoor cycles range from old-fashioned pedal pushers to high-tech models with digital readouts of distance, speed, calories, etc.

The computerized bikes, which are usually found in health clubs, offer varying degrees of difficulty. Since even the first level can be tough for an inexperienced cyclist, you may want to stay with the manual mode.

You may notice that you get tired faster on an indoor cycle than while riding outside. While this is partly due to coasting, which you can't do indoors, I believe it's also psychological. When you're riding outside, there's so much visual and tactile excitement it helps you forget your fatigue.

In cycling, as in many other aerobic sports, you're likely to find that your muscles tire before your heart and lungs do. Just build up slowly, and always do your warm-up and cooldown. Warm-up for biking consists of gentle stretching and slow riding; cooldown is a gentle stretching routine.

Cycling is suitable for all fitness levels. Women with osteoporosis may use recumbent bikes (stationary bikes with back support).

R O W I N G

▶ ▶

Rowing is a non-weight-bearing aerobic activity that benefits the heart and upper body. For rowing to qualify as aerobic, it needs to be done for at least twenty minutes without stopping.

Outdoor rowing options including canoeing, kayaking, crewing, and paddling an old rowboat across a quiet pond. You need a life preserver and a companion to participate in these pastimes. It's an old rule of the sea (and river and lake): Never go out on the water alone.

Most gyms and health clubs have rowing machines, sometimes computerized versions. These should not be used by women with osteoporosis, since the spine is unsupported. If you're not at risk for osteoporosis, you might want to include the rowing machine in an aerobic circuit with the stair machine, treadmill, or cross country ski machine.

Indoor or outdoor rowing is suitable for all fitness levels, but not for women with osteoporosis.

AEROBIC ACTIVITY GUIDELINES

The following charts provide guidelines for the duration and intensity of various aerobic activities for different fitness levels. Once you have determined your fitness level according to the criteria in Chapter 6, you can use the appropriate chart as a menu of aerobic choices. As part of your 4-Week Workout Program, you'll select from this menu to do three to five aerobic sessions each week.

If you are at Fitness Level 1, you may need to start below the recommended duration for the first few weeks or months. Pay attention to your condition and how you feel, and pace yourself carefully. If you have been diagnosed as having osteoporosis, please follow the aerobic recommendations in Chapter 17.

The duration of aerobic dance and step sessions will depend on the class. The duration of other activities can be increased if you have been doing them consistently and qualify as Fitness Level 2 or 3.

The intensity is determined by the percentage of your maximum heart rate, as per the formula in Chapter 6. You should reach this percentage after five to ten minutes of the activity. When you first start out, you may want to use the RPE (Rate of Perceived Exertion) as an alternative method of measuring intensity.

If measuring the intensity is too distracting at first, you can wait until you're more experienced. But be careful to pay attention to your overall comfort level and challenge yourself without overexerting.

LEVEL 1

Aerobic Activity	Duration	Intensity/ Percentage of Maximum Heart Rate
WALK (outside or on treadmill speed 2.8–3.4 mph)	20–30 min.	50–60
BIKE	10–15 min.	50–60
AEROBIC DANCE OR STEP CLASS	Beginner level	50–60
STAIR MACHINE (use level under 4)	10–20 min.	50–60
CROSS-COUNTRY SKI MACHINE	10–15 min.	50–60
SWIMMING (rest between laps)	10–15 min.	50–60
RACQUET SPORTS	20 min.	50–60

LEVEL 2

Aerobic Activity	Duration	Intensity/ Percentage of Maximum Heart Rate
WALK (outside or on treadmill, speed 3.2–3.6 mph)	25–40 min.	60–80
JOG OR WALK/RUN (at 3.6–4.2 mph)	15–20 min.	60–80
BIKE	20–30 min.	60–80
AEROBIC DANCE OR STEP CLASS	Intermediate level	60–80
STAIR MACHINE (use level 4–7)	15–25 min.	60–80
CROSS-COUNTRY SKI MACHINE	10–20 min.	60–80
SWIMMING	15–20 min.	60–80
RACQUET SPORTS	20–30 min.	60–80

AEROBIC ACTIVITY	DURATION	INTENSITY/ PERCENTAGE OF MAXIMUM HEART RATE
WALK (Outside or on treadmill, speed over 3.6 mph)	More than 45 min.	60–80
JOG OR WALK/RUN (at 3.6 mph or over)	20–60 min.	60–80
BIKE	More than 30 min.	60–80
AEROBIC DANCE OR STEP CLASS	Intermediate or advanced level	60–80
STAIR MACHINE (use above level 5)	20–45 min.	60–80
CROSS-COUNTRY SKI MACHINE	20–30 min.	60–80
SWIMMING	20–45 min.	60–80
RACQUET SPORTS	More than 30 min.	60–80

STRENGTH TRAINING
FOR MIDLIFE POWER

After nearly two decades of focusing on aerobic exercise, in the 1990s fitness professionals turned their attention to encouraging strength training, especially for women.

In 1990 the ACSM revised its "Position Stand on the Recommended Quantity and Quality of Exercise for Developing and Maintaining Cardiorespiratory and Muscular Fitness in Healthy Adults" to include the following statement:

"Strength training of a moderate intensity, sufficient to develop and maintain fat-free weight (FFW), should be an integral part of an adult fitness program. One set of eight to twelve repetitions of eight to ten exercises that condition the major muscle groups at least two days a week is the recommended minimum."

Leading experts in the fitness field have also revised their programs and recommendations to include regular strength sessions. Dr. Kenneth Cooper, who fueled the fitness revolution with his classic book *Aerobics*, now prescribes a light weight training program for both adults and children. He acknowledges the merits of strength training in conditioning all the muscles of the body, and encourages people to start this activity early.

For midlife women there are a number of compelling reasons to add strength training to their weekly routine. The foremost reason is the need to strengthen the muscles attached to the bones to help prevent or to manage osteoporosis and reduce the risk of fracture.

Strength training can also reduce the risk of back problems and injuries. It can help you lose fat, firm your body, and improve your figure. And, according to William Evans, Ph.D., it can even offset some of the symptoms of aging.

MUSCLE STRENGTH AS A BIOMARKER

▶ ▶ ▶ ▶ ▶ ▶ ▶ ▶ ▶ ▶

In his pioneering book *Biomarkers: The 10 Keys to Prolonging Vitality* (coauthored by Dr. Irwin H. Rosenberg with Jacqueline Thompson), Dr. Evans offers a fitness and nutrition self-help program to improve the ten markers of biological aging. Biomarker 1 is muscle mass and Biomarker 2 is strength.

Dr. Evans cites studies that indicate the average person's lean body mass and strength declines with age, especially after the age of forty-five. This muscle loss has a negative effect on other biomarkers and can result in a slower metabolism, an increase in body fat, a decline in aerobic capacity, reduced blood-sugar tolerance, and loss in bone density. Since muscle strength influences so many barometers of aging, Dr. Evans's Biomarker Program emphasizes rebuilding and maintaining strength.

Studies at the USDA Human Nutrition Research Center on Aging (HNRCA) at Tufts University found that when older people participated in a strength-training program, hypertrophy (muscle growth) was dramatic. In fact, the degree of muscle growth was as high as would be expected in young people doing the same amount of exercise. These studies prove a person is never too old to build muscle and offset the muscle loss of aging.

LOSE FAT AND BUILD MUSCLE

▶ ▶ ▶ ▶ ▶ ▶ ▶ ▶ ▶ ▶

It's a sad but true fact of life that many women find their waists thickening and their bodies becoming less toned as they age. Strength training, along with healthy nutrition, is a primary way to counteract the dreaded "middle-age spread."

There's an expression I use to motivate clients: *You have to lift weight to lose weight.* To be more specific, while strength training may not lead to weight loss on the scale, it is likely to result in fat loss and a slimmer appearance.

Strength training helps you shape your body into the shape you want. The loss of body fat and increase in lean muscle tissue can noticeably enhance the way you look and feel. After a few months of regular weight training, you may notice that your stomach is flatter and your waist is more defined. Your breasts may appear firmer and higher as the underlying pectoral muscles become stronger. Your entire body can become firmer and tighter.

Strength-training workouts also rev up your metabolic rate, which means you'll burn more calories during all activities, even sleeping. In midlife, most women begin to lose muscle, and for every pound of muscle lost, your resting metabolic rate drops by nearly fifty calories a day. This process can be reversed as your metabolic rate rises when you build muscle.

A study of ten postmenopausal women at Tufts University found that after six weeks of training the group had lost twenty pounds, most of it fat. They had also raised their metabolism between 10 and 15 percent. The women burned an additional fifty calories for every pound of muscle they had gained.

POSTURE AND PRESENCE

Posture has a powerful influence on how others perceive us, and on how we feel about ourselves. A slumped posture can cause a woman to look and feel insignificant, weak, and lethargic. An uplifted posture says to the world: Here I am, proud and powerful! Mature women with beautiful posture are noticed, respected, and admired.

Many women who want to improve their posture don't have the muscle to maintain it. Good posture requires strength—to keep your spine elongated, shoulders down and back, and neck long. Strength training gives you the muscle to maintain elegantly erect posture.

The significance of posture goes beyond appearance. Posture affects your energy level, since it can either restrict or facilitate blood flow. Good posture also reduces your risk of headaches, backaches, and painful spinal misalignments.

POSITIVE POWER

Midlife is a time when many women achieve new levels of power in their professional lives. With strength training, you can match and fuel your professional power with an exciting surge of physical power. Here's what some midlife women have said about their muscle strength work:

> "Getting strong has made me more secure and confident in so many different areas of my life. It's great not to feel weak and helpless anymore."

> "Strength training helps me cope with so many everyday things—carrying the groceries, holding my granddaughter, cleaning my house, everything!"

> "I do a lot of business traveling, and now that I'm stronger I enjoy being able to handle my own luggage easily. I always book hotels that have gyms."

"Strength training makes me feel stronger mentally as well as physically. I feel more powerful and confident when I'm negotiating a business deal."

THE DEFINITION OF STRENGTH TRAINING

▸ ▸ ▸ ▸ ▸ ▸ ▸ ▸ ▸ ▸ ▸

Many people confuse strength training with bodybuilding or weightlifting. These sports are actually advanced or extreme forms of strength training, and far different from the strength training exercises in the Strength Training Routines.

Strength training, which is also called muscle-strength/endurance exercise, involves working individual muscle groups. This can be done by using your own body weight as resistance, or an outside force such as weights, bands, tubes, water, or equipment in health clubs.

Strength training works by two basic principles: overload and progressive resistance.

The overload principle means a muscle has to be stressed and worked close to its force-generating capacity to increase in strength. Basically, for a muscle to grow in strength, it needs to do more work than usual. In strength training, this is done by lifting your own body weight or an outside weight for resistance.

The second principle, progressive resistance, refers to the need to increase overload to continue building strength. This involves gradually adding weight and increasing the number of repetitions and sets of the exercises you do.

Repetition of strength exercises changes your muscles at the fiber and neurological levels. This increases strength, endurance, reaction time, and force—the training effect.

TYPES OF STRENGTH TRAINING

▸ ▸ ▸ ▸ ▸ ▸ ▸ ▸ ▸ ▸ ▸

There are three basic forms of strength-training exercises: isotonic, isometric, and isokinetic.

ISOTONIC EXERCISES are performed by raising or lowering a weight through the joint's full range of motion. Although the weight is constant, the resistance level fluctuates throughout the lift, becoming easier toward the end.

Isotonic exercises are typically done with free weights or machines such as Nautilus or Universal. Bodybuilding and weightlifting are more intense forms of isotonic exercise.

When you're starting out, it's helpful to have a trainer demonstrate how to use the isotonic equipment. If you learn to use the equipment carefully and start with a modest routine, you may find great satisfaction and results with this type of workout.

ISOMETRIC EXERCISES involve contracting the muscle and holding it in a position for a few seconds. Isometric exercises were very popular in the 1950s and 1960s. Development in the fitness world has shown that isometrics are best combined with other forms of strength training.

ISOKINETIC EXERCISES are usually done on equipment that utilizes a hydraulic form of resistance. This creates a constant level of resistance at a fixed rate of contraction throughout the joint's full range of motion. It is generally used in clinical or rehabilitation settings.

Using your own body weight as resistance is another form of strength training. For example, in sit-ups and pushups gravity and the weight of your own body provide resistance to strengthen muscles.

STRENGTH TRAINING ROUTINE

▶ ▶ ▶ ▶ ▶ ▶ ▶ ▶ ▶ ▶ ▶

The Strength Training Routine combines a basic warm-up with a series of strength-training exercises and a cooldown in four easy-to-follow routines. These are designed to be thorough without being cruel, and provide the gain without the pain.

The routine meets the two basic criteria for building muscle strength and endurance: the overload principle and progressive resistance. The overload is achieved through lifting your body weight and using hand and ankle weights in some exercises. The progressive resistance comes as you continue to do the routine and gradually add weights, sets, and repetitions over a period of months.

The routine also meets another requirement of a successful strength-training program: balance. Balance is necessary to reduce the risk of injury and have a symmetrical appearance.

Balanced muscles work together to keep stress off the joints. For instance, if you have lower back pain the exercise prescription is to strengthen your abdominal muscles and stretch your hamstrings (back of thighs) so these muscles can support your back.

A strength-training routine should fatigue the major muscles first and then the smaller muscles. It should challenge the front and back of your body equally. It should work different muscle groups on different days. Since strength training is site specific—it develops the specific muscles being worked—you need a systematic and comprehensive routine.

All these considerations can be complicated. That's why I've done the work for you—all you need to do is the routine! If you do the Strength Training Routine two days a week (with at least one day of rest between each session), you can be assured that your strength-training program is balanced and safe.

While you're doing the routine, or any other strength-training exercise, remember to *keep breathing*. Although this may sound like a silly reminder, it's easy to hold your breath when lifting weight or exerting yourself. Since strength training increases blood pressure slightly, you don't want to exacerbate this condition by holding your breath.

The rule in strength training is simple: *Exhale on the exertion.* Generally, this means inhaling on the lengthening motion or lowering of the weight, and exhaling on the lift.

When you schedule your strength workouts, be sure to have a day of rest in between. Since strength training causes microscopic tears in muscle fibers, you need that day of recovery between workouts for repair.

If you're not accustomed to strength training, you may experience some aches and pains during the first few sessions. You may feel fine immediately after a workout, then sore in the next day or two, a phenomenon called DOMS (Delayed Onset of Muscle Soreness).

If you're very sore, wait forty-eight hours before resuming exercise. You may want to do gentle stretching during this recovery period. If any sharp pain or continued soreness results, see your health care professional before continuing your workout program.

BODYBUILDING AND WEIGHTLIFTING
▸ ▸ ▸ ▸ ▸ ▸ ▸ ▸ ▸ ▸ ▸

The Strength Training Routine will firm and tone your body. You may notice development in your shoulders, arms, and legs, a firming of your abdomen, buttocks, and thighs, and other subtle changes. You will *not* develop large, bulky muscles from doing the routine alone.

Many midlife women start with basic strength-training exercises and find the power surge exciting. They want to take training a step further and delve into bodybuilding.

The goal of bodybuilding is to develop and display heavy, symmetrical, defined muscles. This is achieved through the use of free-standing weights such as barbells and dumbbells, and isotonic machines.

Although bodybuilders do spend a great deal of time lifting weights, their sport is technically different than weightlifting, which involves competitions to lift the heaviest weights. Bodybuilding competitions are judged on the size, shape, symmetry, and definition of the muscles.

Bodybuilding has become increasingly popular for women, and there are even seniors divisions in competitions. Whether or not you decide to pursue bodybuilding is a personal decision. My only recommendation is don't get carried away and risk harming yourself.

Avoid anabolic steroids and hormones for bodybuilding. Work with a qualified trainer who respects your body's limitations. And remember: A midlife woman's power comes from her mind, not just her muscles.

THE PLEASURE OF FLEXIBILITY AND RELAXATION

"I think stretching and relaxation exercises are crucially important, since the more you maintain flexibility through stretching, the more you tend to offset the diminished flexibility we thought was due to aging. Much of what we thought was due to aging is really due to disuse."

—ELIZABETH LEE VLIET, M.D.

Stretching is a reward for your body and soul. It can be the icing on the cake after a strenuous workout or a welcome relief after a stressful day on the job. Yet stretching is more than a pleasure and its benefits go far beyond relaxation.

Flexibility and strength complement each other. Flexibility is the flip side of strength and lets you build muscles that are lengthened as well as strong. When you're strengthening one muscle you're usually stretching another. For example, when you're strengthening the back of your legs, you're stretching the front; and when you're strengthening your abdominals you're stretching your back.

Stretching counteracts the stiffness that often creeps up in midlife and allows you to feel loose and limber once again. It enhances coordination and agility and gives you a wider range of movement. It reduces the risk of injuries from both everyday activities and exercise.

Stretching is a wonderful way to get in touch with the intimate connection between your body and mind. When you settle down to stretch you can feel the areas that are tight from the physical and emotional stress of your day.

If you breathe deeply and relax into your stretching exercises, they can help you to be more flexible mentally as well as physically. Stretching can open up a sense of being calm and centered.

FLEXIBILITY

▸ ▸ ▸ ▸ ▸ ▸ ▸ ▸ ▸ ▸ ▸

Flexibility is the ability to move a joint through its full range of motion. Many midlife women complain of loss of flexibility and a general stiffness in their muscles and joints. Yet this is not an inevitable result of aging; it is largely due to inactivity.

Without regular stretching and other exercise, muscles tighten. The end result is a lack of flexibility and a feeling of stiffness, along with vulnerability to back pain and injuries.

Flexibility exercises counteract this loss by stretching your muscle fibers. Gentle stretching lengthens your muscle fibers and facilitates the movement of joints the muscles control. Stretching can soothe pain caused by tight muscles and injuries. It can also release pressure on the nerves and alleviate ailments such as tension headaches and neck and back pain.

THE SAFE WAY TO STRETCH

▸ ▸ ▸ ▸ ▸ ▸ ▸ ▸ ▸ ▸ ▸

There are several ways to stretch a muscle. In the 4-Week Workout Program we use static stretching. This involves slowly lengthening a muscle to the point of tension, then holding the position for ten to thirty seconds. With static stretching there is less chance of stretching beyond your limits and risking injury or soreness.

Years ago you may have taken frenetic exercise classes that included bouncing stretches. Now, fitness professionals generally frown on bouncing because it activates the stretch reflex. This is when stretching a tight muscle activates the nervous system and your brain sends a signal to stop stretching. It's one of your body's mechanisms to protect you from injury.

In strength training, we aim to do a certain number of sets and repetitions. In flexibility, the goal is different: sustained holding of the stretch. Flexibility requires patience and relaxation to achieve results.

Before you stretch, your muscles should be warm. This doesn't necessarily mean you need to do a full aerobic routine; the warm-up stretching sequence before the Strength Training Routine or ten minutes of walking in place should do.

Find a quiet, comfortable place to stretch, with an exercise mat or carpet. Wear clothing that allows you full range of motion.

Exhale as you move slowly and smoothly into a stretch. You should stretch until you feel mild tension, then release slightly and hold the position for ten to thirty seconds to allow the muscle to lengthen. Keep breathing and concentrate on relaxing and lengthening as you hold the stretch. Move out of the stretch gently.

Begin by stretching the major, large muscles first; then stretch the supporting, smaller muscles. The Flexibility Cooldown sequence, which is done after the Strength Training Routine, follows this pattern. This stretching routine can be done after every aerobic or strength-training session, and used as an overall "stretcher" between workouts.

A special note for women with osteoporosis: While it is important that you stretch on a regular basis, your flexibility exercises will be modified. You should not do any forward flexion (bending from the waist) or twisting movements. Warm-up and Flexibility Cooldown stretches that meet these guidelines are included in Chapter 17.

STRETCHING THROUGH YOUR DAY
▸ ▸ ▸ ▸ ▸ ▸ ▸ ▸ ▸ ▸

If you're a typically busy midlife woman, you're probably interested in how to incorporate exercise into your already hectic day. While you need to set aside time for flexibility exercises (particularly after aerobics and strength training) you can also give yourself a bonus by adding stretching here and there during your day. These stretching breaks will relieve tension and give you more energy for all your activities.

Hold each stretch for ten to thirty seconds unless otherwise stated. Breathe and relax as you stretch; don't bounce.

STRETCHES TO DO IN BED

1. Put your pillow aside and move down toward the foot of the bed. Stretch your arms overhead and legs out. Inhale, then exhale as you stretch your right arm up and right leg down, lengthening the whole right side of your body. Inhale as you release. Exhale as you stretch your left arm and left leg. Alternate, stretching three times on each side.

2. Lying on your back, bend your knees and exhale as you gently hug them to your body. Circle your knees slowly in both directions to stretch out your lower back.

3. Sitting up in bed cross-legged, slowly move your head to the right and to the left three times. Shrug your shoulders up and down gently. Place your hands on your shoulders and circle your elbows forward three times; back three times.

STRETCHES TO DO IN YOUR OFFICE

1. In your chair, exhale as you slowly lower your head, round your back, and bend at the waist so that chest and head hang over your legs. Breathe and release. Roll up slowly, one vertebra at a time.

2. In your chair, clasp your hands and exhale as you stretch your arms up toward the ceiling. Hold the stretch with your palms facing the ceiling. Open your arms and lower them to the side, bringing your hands behind your chair. Hold on to the back of your chair and lean forward to stretch your back. Slowly release.

3. In your chair, exhale as you slowly twist to the right, placing your left hand on your right knee for leverage. Press your right shoul-

der back as you hold this position, feeling the stretch in your back. Repeat on the other side, twisting to the left.

4. Stand up. Clasp your hands behind your back. Lift arms away from body while keeping elbows straight. Hold and breathe deeply for thirty seconds, then release.

THE STRESS RESPONSE
▸ ▸ ▸ ▸ ▸ ▸ ▸ ▸ ▸ ▸ ▸

Most midlife women face a great deal of stress, juggling jobs and the demands of managing a home and a personal life. Further stress can result from caring for aging parents; dealing with teenage children or the empty nest syndrome; and issues with husbands, partners, or being single. Hormonal fluctuations, hot flashes, and other symptoms of menopause can make it difficult to cope with stress.

Obviously, some stress is healthy to keep your life challenging and interesting. It's virtually impossible to have a stress-free life. The goal is not to eliminate stress completely, but to learn to maintain your health and well-being despite the stresses of life.

You can cope with stress overload by using this three-pronged approach:

▸ Evaluate your lifestyle to see where stress can be reduced. Seek the help of friends and family, support groups, and therapy if you think it is appropriate.
▸ Exercise on a regular basis to counteract the effects of stress.
▸ Practice techniques to induce relaxation.

Stress has far more than emotional effects; it induces a series of physiological responses. In reaction to intense or prolonged stress your body reacts with a fight or flight response. This is a survival response dating back to the time when stress involved a physical threat: perhaps a wild animal entering the cave or barbaric hordes storming into the village. Now, although stress is often emotionally rather than physically threatening, the body's instinctual response remains the same.

The reactive state induced by stress can include these changes:

▸ Increase in heartbeat
▸ Rapid, shallow breathing
▸ Rise in blood pressure
▸ Rise in blood sugar level
▸ Muscle tension
▸ Increase in blood flow to the brain and major muscles

In the modern world we have little physical release for these stress reactions. You can't work off muscle tension by vigorously clubbing an infuriating spouse or impossible teenager. You can't utilize the increase in blood flow to run like the wind when your supervisor gives you an unreasonable deadline. Without any outlet, the biochemical reaction to stress can cause a number of ailments.

The most effective way to counteract the physical effects of the stress response is to evoke conscious relaxation. This is different than the relaxation that stems from having a glass of wine with your best friend or reading a trashy novel, pleasant as these activities may be. Conscious relaxation involves specific practices and physiological changes.

Dr. Herbert Benson, a cardiologist and a leading researcher in the field of psychoneuroimmunology, coined the term "the relaxation response" to describe the process and benefits of conscious relaxation. In his classic book of the same name, he gives a simple method based on meditation to elicit this response, along with an explanation of its effects, which can include:

▸ Decreased activity of the sympathetic nervous system
▸ Slower heart and respiratory rates
▸ Lower blood pressure
▸ Release of muscle tension

Conscious relaxation methods include deep breathing, meditation, autogenic training, progressive relaxation, yoga, and biofeedback. Numerous studies have indicated that practicing a relaxation technique for twenty minutes a day has dramatic physiological and emotional benefits.

An added benefit of relaxation methods is their ability to diminish hot flashes in some women. A 1984 project by researchers at the Lafayette Clinic and Wayne State University studied the effect of relaxation practices (progressive muscle relaxation and biofeedback) on hot flash frequency in fourteen women. Symptom diaries kept by the participants reported a significant reduction in frequency of hot flashes and a longer delay between exposure to heat stress and hot flash onset.

It should be noted that *consistent* practice of relaxation methods is needed to have an effect on hot flashes. According to Dr. Alice Domar, a health psychologist who works with Dr. Benson, "It's important to do a relaxation technique every day for the carryover effect. You start feeling better all day. It's the carryover effect that leads to the decrease in hot flashes."

Many women feel that a daily dose of relaxation practice is indispensable to their sense of well-being. Others practice intermittently and use conscious relaxation as a healing tool in especially stressful times.

As with exercise, the best way to learn about the benefits of the relaxation response is to experience them. Some relaxation techniques, such as meditation and yoga, require practice, while others are as simple as breathing like a sleeping baby.

DEEP BREATHING

Deep breathing, which is also called diaphragmatic or yoga breathing, is a simple method for evoking conscious relaxation. This type of breathing is done by expanding the abdomen and lungs completely so the diaphragm (the muscle that separates the chest cavity from the abdomen) lowers to allow lung expansion. It may sound complicated, but it's the natural way for a baby or someone in a relaxed state of sleep to breathe.

To practice deep breathing, lie down on your bed or on an exercise mat or carpet. Loosen any restrictive clothing you might have on. Close your eyes and place your hands on your abdomen.

Deep breathing is done through the nose, not the mouth. Begin by exhaling slowly and completely. Then inhale slowly through your nose, filling your abdomen with breath. You should feel your abdomen expand under your fingers. Continue to inhale, filling up your rib cage and then your chest. Exhale slowly and completely. Do this four or five times on the first session.

Once you've become accustomed to deep breathing, you can turn it into a simple relaxation technique. Inhale slowly for a count of eight; hold for a count of four, exhale slowly for a count of eight. You can do this for ten to twenty minutes, to clear your mind and elicit relaxation.

Deep breathing is also a technique you can utilize in your everyday life. The next time you're feeling stressed or overloaded, notice how you're breathing. Then exhale completely through your nose and begin slowly to fill yourself up with relaxing breath: abdomen, rib cage, lungs. If you focus on this for even five minutes, you'll find it relaxing and refreshing. Deep breathing is nature's tranquilizer, available for our use anytime, anywhere.

AUTOGENIC TRAINING AND PROGRESSIVE RELAXATION

Autogenic training and progressive relaxation are techniques to release muscle tension, facilitate relaxation, and teach you control over your body. They are performed by focusing on each part of your body to induce muscle release.

Many women find it helpful to use relaxation audiotapes, which feature a calm voice that guides you through a step-by-step process. You can also make your own relaxation tape by recording the following instructions. Or you can memorize the instructions and silently "talk" yourself through the relaxation sessions.

AUTOGENIC TRAINING EXERCISE

1. Lie down, close your eyes, and practice deep breathing for at least five breaths.

2. Bring your attention to each part of your body in the following sequence, and say to yourself these suggestive phrases. Stay focused on one body part until you actually feel the sensation you are evoking; then move on to the next area:

My right arm feels heavy and warm.

My left arm feels heavy and warm.

My right leg feels heavy and warm.

My left leg feels heavy and warm.

My abdomen and chest feel relaxed and warm.

My breathing is gentle and my heartbeat is calm.

My back and shoulders are heavy and warm.

My neck and head are heavy and cool.

3. Take several moments to enjoy the relaxation and float. You may want to repeat positive affirmations to yourself during this time.

4. When you are ready, count slowly backwards from three to one. Then flex your hands and feet, open your eyes, and stretch your body gently. After a minute or two you can rise up slowly, feeling relaxed and refreshed.

PROGRESSIVE RELAXATION EXERCISE

1. Lie down, close your eyes, and practice deep breathing for at least five breaths.

2. Bring your attention to each part of your body in the following sequence. Stay focused on one body part until you actually feel the sensation you are evoking; then move on to the next part.

Inhale and tighten your entire right arm by making a fist and lifting your arm. Exhale and let your arm flop down and sink, relaxed. Repeat with your left arm.

Inhale and tighten your entire right leg by pointing your toes and lifting your leg a few inches into the air. Exhale and let your leg release down and sink to the ground. Repeat with your left leg.

Inhale into your abdomen; hold and tighten your stomach; exhale and release. Inhale and hold your breath in your chest; exhale and release.

Inhale and raise your shoulders in a shrug; exhale and release, opening your shoulder blades.

Inhale and lift your head about six inches off the ground. Exhale and slowly release. Let your head sink into the ground and relax your neck.

Inhale and tighten your face by puckering your lips and squinting your eyes. Exhale and allow your face to expand and completely relax.

3. Take several moments to enjoy the relaxation and float. You may want to repeat positive affirmations to yourself during this interlude. If there are any tight spots in your body, gently massage them.

4. When you are ready, count slowly backwards from three to one. Then flex your hands and feet, open your eyes, and gently stretch your body. After a minute or so you can rise up slowly, feeling relaxed and refreshed.

RELAXATION TECHNIQUES AND EXERCISE
▶ ▶ ▶ ▶ ▶ ▶ ▶ ▶ ▶ ▶

"We advise women to evoke the relaxation response while they're exercising. Focus on the cadence of the feet or the breath while you're working."

—ALICE DOMAR, PH.D.

In a perfect world, women would have time for a strength-training or aerobic workout and a twenty-minute relaxation session five days a week. But in reality, it's often difficult to find time for both.

One way around this barrier is to practice conscious relaxation while you work out. This is possible in many forms of exercise, particularly rhythmic activities such as walking, running, swimming, and biking.

You can achieve a relaxation effect by clearing your mind and focusing on your breath, a body part, or a key word or phrase. One of the most natural techniques is to concentrate on your breath. You can also count "one-two" with every step as you walk or run. If you swim, counting laps can be a form of meditation.

Since it's not easy to clear your mind of other thoughts and focus, it's helpful first to practice relaxation methods when you're quiet and still. Then you can add a new dimension to some of your exercise sessions with relaxation techniques.

Yoga involves stretching, relaxation, and much more. It encompasses an astonishing variety of practices for the development of the mind and body and can be done on many levels.

Yoga evolved in India thousands of years ago and has now spread around the globe. Many of the benefits of yoga, which the ancient yogis may have sensed instinctively, have been proven in scientific studies. These include benefits for all the major systems of the body: respiratory, nervous, digestive, muscular, and hormonal.

Yoga practice enhances flexibility and muscular development and elicits the relaxation response. If practiced religiously, it can bring spiritual development and enlightenment.

The word "yoga" is based on the Sanskrit word for union or joining. This refers to the ultimate goal of yoga, which is the joining of the physical, mental, and spiritual selves and, on a higher level, the union of human beings and the Creator. The advanced study of yoga involves moral living, good works, meditation, sobriety, and vegetarianism. But many people practice yoga simply as a way to stretch, relax, and feel terrific.

The most familiar form of yoga in the West is Hatha yoga. Ideally, this is a path to a greater spiritual realization through mental and physical control of the mind and body. This is achieved through meditation, breathing exercises, and *asanas*, which are the poses or postures.

These postures form the basis of many yoga classes in the U.S., where yoga is taught everywhere from Y's, gyms, and continuing education centers to yoga centers and *ashrams*. You can also learn yoga from videotapes and books. However, at some point it's wise to work with a teacher who can give you advice and inspiration.

If you would like to learn yoga, you'll find a wealth of options in many areas of the country. Yoga teachers vary widely in style, from those who are spiritually oriented to those who focus on yoga as exercise. Try to watch a class or take a trial session before committing to a series of classes. Look for an instructor who teaches carefully and helps students avoid injury. A yoga teacher should be patient, compassionate, knowledgeable, and encouraging.

One wonderful quality of yoga is you're never too old to learn it or practice it. If practiced carefully and correctly, it is a gentle and generally safe form of exercise for midlife women. It's ideal for maintaining a sense of balance during midlife and menopause, reducing anxiety, and enhancing mood. And it can be practiced well into old age. Many devotees find that yoga actually delays the symptoms of aging and allows them to remain flexible, vigorous, and positive.

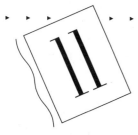

NUTRITION FOR MIDLIFE HEALTH

"For anyone who is concerned about health, the goal is more plant, less animal; more whole, less processed; move more, sit less."

—SHARON AKABAS, PH.D.

Assistant Professor of Nutrition and Education
Columbia University Teachers College

An active lifestyle and a balanced diet work synergistically to help you stay healthy throughout midlife. Any exercise program, including the 4-Week Workout Program, will be more successful when supported by sound nutrition.

The 4-Week Workout Program emphasizes eating for energy rather than immediate weight loss. But if you eat modest portions of nutritious foods and increase your exercise, you will likely lose excess weight. You'll gain muscle and lose fat as you firm and tone your body.

EATING FOR ENERGY

▸ ▸ ▸ ▸ ▸ ▸ ▸ ▸ ▸ ▸ ▸

"Food is fuel, not a fattening enemy."

—NANCY CLARK, M.S., R.D.

Director of Nutrition Services at Sports Medicine Brookline, Massachusetts

Instead of thinking about what you should *not* eat, try an experiment: For the first month of the Workout Program, focus on what you *should* eat to fuel your body for exercise. Just as a car works better on high-quality fuel, so does your body. The optimal fuel for the human body is food that comes from nature, in as close to its natural form as possible.

Foods that enhance energy and health include:

▸ Vegetables
▸ Fruits
▸ Whole grains
▸ Nuts, seeds, and legumes

Certain types of fish and limited amounts of dairy products, chicken, turkey, and eggs, can also be part of a balanced diet. The foods and beverages to limit or avoid are those with high amounts of animal fat, sugar, food additives, and caffeine.

If you have a lifelong habit of eating a lot of refined sugar, highly processed foods, and meat, this pattern may be deeply ingrained. And caffeine is known to be as addictive as many drugs. It's helpful to seek out books, programs, and people for support in changing these habits.

What has worked for many of my clients is to change gradually. If you decide to overhaul your diet completely, you may feel overwhelmed and end up making no changes whatsoever. An approach that is often more successful is to start with small changes and gradually shift your diet toward natural, fresh foods.

For example, try taking fruit to work to have as a snack instead of a donut. Or drink fruit juice mixed with seltzer instead of sugary soda. Or use whole grain bread and brown rice to replace white bread and refined white rice. You could also choose whole grain cereals sweetened with fruit juice instead of highly processed cereals with high sugar content. Start reading labels in the supermarket and avoid items with food additives.

During the Workout Program, you're going to be adventurous by trying different types of exercise. At the same time, you can experiment with your diet.

Taste a tofuburger with tahini sauce instead of a hamburger. Buy different types of vegetables from a Latin or Asian market. Stock your fridge with an exotic fruit salad to nibble when you crave something sweet. Order steamed vegetables over brown rice from a Chinese takeout instead of pork fried rice. Be creative and open yourself up to the diverse world of healthy, delicious food.

There are many other ways to make whole foods a natural part of your life. Here are some choices to try—in moderation:

- Try to buy organic produce whenever possible. Many markets have organic sections or specially marked products.
- Prepare little "nibble bags" of seeds, nuts, and dried fruit to take to work for snacks. Be aware that although nuts and seeds are healthy, they are highly caloric and should be eaten in small amounts.
- Lightly steam vegetables or eat them raw instead of boiled or sautéed.
- Make salads more interesting by using a variety of leafy greens (not iceberg lettuce, which is low in nutritive value).
- Keep a bowl or plastic bag full of washed, raw vegetables in your fridge for munchies.

- Buy a juicer to prepare super-high-energy drinks for yourself.
- Increase fiber by selecting cereals, pastas, and bread made with whole grains.

ENERGY EATING: WHEN, WHERE, AND HOW MUCH

▸ ▸ ▸ ▸ ▸ ▸ ▸ ▸ ▸ ▸ ▸

It's not just what you eat but *when* you eat that affects your energy level. For many people it's best to eat five or six *small* meals a day instead of three large ones. This provides a steady flow of nutrients without taxing your digestive system. It can also prevent blood sugar level fluctuations that leave you feeling tired and drained.

Nutritionists often recommend having breakfast be your largest meal of the day and dinner the smallest as a health and weight-loss strategy. This is sensible because you have the entire day to work off your morning meal, while the period after dinner is often sedentary. However, in the real world, dinner is a social meal, and this plan may not be practical. You can modify this advice by eating a light, early dinner several nights of the week.

Whenever you eat, sit down, relax, and eat *consciously*. Unconscious eating is often a major cause of weight gain. If you eat on the run or at the counter, you won't feel nourished and are likely to eat too much of the wrong foods. If you sit down and focus on the taste and texture of what you're eating, you'll get more satisfaction from it.

Try not to confuse boredom or tension with hunger. If you need a break from work or children or whatever, try an exercise session, a glass of water, a relaxation technique, or even a short nap. Take a deep breath and consider what you really need instead of automatically going for a snack. If it is a snack you truly want and need, choose one consciously and enjoy it.

If you're concerned about weight loss, beware that even healthy, high energy foods can put on pounds if you eat too much. Excess carbohydrates can be stored as fat. *Portion control is the key.* Modest portions also maintain your energy level and keep you from feeling weighed down and sluggish. And if you sit down to eat consciously and slowly, you'll feel satisfied even if your plate isn't heaped high.

WATER, WATER, WATER

▸ ▸ ▸ ▸ ▸ ▸ ▸ ▸ ▸ ▸ ▸

Water is a tremendous tool for keeping your energy up and your weight down. It's the most essential nutrient of life—and it has zero calories! Yet despite all its benefits, few women drink enough water on a daily basis. A basic guideline is to drink six to eight glasses of water a day; one glass for each twenty pounds you weigh.

Drinking plenty of water cleans out your system and discourages overeating. Staying well hydrated also helps relieve constipation, a complaint that sometimes worsens with menopause. Increasing your water intake is recommended for everything from detoxification to keeping your skin fresh and youthful. If there is a Fountain of Youth, it must be flowing with fresh, clean water.

Since many public water supplies have purification systems of questionable efficiency, you may want to invest in a home water cooler, a high-quality filter, or large jugs of spring water. A good way to remember to drink enough water is to carry a small plastic water bottle with you and refill it throughout the day.

Some women try to limit their water intake to keep their weight down or to avoid looking bloated. But bloating can be a sign of dehydration and of your body holding on to its deficient supply of water. If you get in the habit of drinking plenty of water, you'll find it actually helps you stay trim by cleansing your system and giving you the hydration needed for energy and exercise.

EATING AND EXERCISING

▶ ▶ ▶ ▶ ▶ ▶ ▶ ▶ ▶ ▶

You may remember when you were a kid there was a mother's rule that you shouldn't go swimming until an hour after eating or you'd get a cramp. Of course, all us kids dove into the water right after polishing off ice cream bars and felt fine anyway.

The moral is that there are no hard and fast rules about eating and exercising except to listen to your body and use your common sense. You don't want to run off to step class an hour after eating a spaghetti and meatball dinner, but it may be okay if you had a yogurt or half a bagel.

It's recommended to wait two hours after eating or drinking anything before you do yoga. You can probably go for a walk at a moderate pace soon after a modest meal. It all depends on what and how much you eat, and the type and intensity of the exercise. Keep in mind your personal metabolism and digestive system, and the available bathrooms where you'll be exercising.

Unless you go in for marathon running, serious hiking, or other exceptional activities, there's no need to carbo-load before a workout. But you shouldn't be starving and thinking about food during the session either. If you haven't had an opportunity to eat for a while and want to have a banana or a piece of bread shortly before a moderate aerobic or strength workout, help yourself. Also consider what you ate and drank the day before, since this is the fuel you'll be primarily using.

Regarding specific fuel for exercise, a nutritious diet with plenty of water is sufficient for moderate workouts under normal circumstances. Fuel bars and electrolyte replacement drinks are more appropriate for marathon running, long-distance hiking and biking, or any activity done for longer than ninety minutes.

Don't fool yourself into thinking that you need additional calories because you're exercising more frequently, unless you're going into serious training. Many women sabotage their weight loss goals by "working up an appetite" through exercise and then overindulging.

Exercise helps with metabolic factors and burning fat, but to lose weight you still need to create a calorie deficit: *You need to burn off more calories than you consume.*

Low-fat doesn't necessarily mean low-calorie. Eating large quantities of pasta, rice, and bread can put on or keep on extra weight, even if you exercise regularly. Nutritionists are now turning away from the low-fat, high-carbohydrate credo and emphasizing fruits, vegetables, and moderate carbohydrates.

NUTRITION AND HERBS FOR MENOPAUSE

▶ ▶ ▶ ▶ ▶ ▶ ▶ ▶ ▶ ▶ ▶

"Some people may notice that particular foods or situations trigger hot flashes. For these individuals, avoiding such foods may reduce the hot flashes. If offending situations are unavoidable, at least women can be prepared for the ensuing hot flash."

— FREDI KRONENBERG, PH.D.

Director of Rosenthal Center for Alternative/Complementary Medicine, College of Physicians and Surgeons of Columbia University

Eating for energy can reduce many of the symptoms of menopause, such as fatigue, depression, and weight gain. Small, light meals consisting of fruits, vegetables, whole grains, and protein can help you feel better throughout the transition and afterwards. Menopause can mark a passage into a healthier way of eating.

During menopause it's advisable to eliminate or limit consumption of caffeine, alcohol, and refined sugar. These substances can aggravate anxiety, fatigue, mood swings, and in some cases, hot flashes.

The relationship between food and hot flashes is still under debate. Some women notice that caffeine, alcohol, fatty food, or heavy spices seem to trigger their hot flashes. Most experts believe hot flash triggers are highly individual.

During menopause, and at any time of life, a diet that provides all the essential vitamins in their natural forms is the ideal. If you suspect that you're not getting enough vitamins from food sources, you may want to supplement them. A multivitamin supplement should include the Recommended Daily Allowance (RDA) of vitamins A, C, and E, and the B complex, which can help with various menopausal symptoms.

Herbs and foods that contain substances similar to estrogen and progesterone are also used to relieve the symptoms of menopause. Other herbal remedies for menopausal symptoms include relaxing teas and Chinese herbs.

If you're interested in herbal remedies, it's wise to seek the advise of a qualified herbalist, nutritionist, or a doctor practicing natural medicine. Herbs are potent substances that can be remarkably beneficial, but they can also have side effects, and you should have the guidance of a knowledgeable practitioner.

Women face an increased risk of two major conditions after menopause: heart disease and osteoporosis. Nutrition is instrumental in preventing both these ailments.

The nutritional advice for preventing heart disease is well known and is the same for men and women. The objective is to keep your cholesterol level down with a diet low in animal fats. You should also try to maintain a healthy weight, which means limiting consumption of sugar and dairy products, and eating moderate portions of protein and carbohydrates.

To prevent osteoporosis and maintain bone density, calcium and vitamin D are required. The National Osteoporosis Foundation's *Physician's Resource Manual* states: "Adequate calcium intake—above the threshold—is absolutely required for bone health, normal bone growth and maturation, and prevention of excessive bone loss with advancing age. The key issue is not 'calcium' versus 'no calcium,' it is how much calcium and what form is recommended."

The RDA for calcium intake is 800 mg for adults. However, concern about osteoporosis has led to the development of new standards.

In 1989, the National Institutes of Health Consensus Development Conference on Optimal Calcium Intake presented these recommendations for daily calcium intake:

Premenopausal women ages 25–50	1,000 mg
Menopausal and postmenopausal women taking estrogen	1,000 mg
Menopausal and postmenopausal women *not* taking estrogen	1,500 mg

There are certain medical conditions, such as calcium-containing kidney stones, that may contraindicate high calcium intake. Check with your doctor about these concerns before increasing your calcium intake.

Many women are confused by the question of calcium derived from food versus calcium derived from supplements. There are a number of individualized factors involved, including calcium absorption, weight control, and food sensitivities. However, the general consensus is that calcium derived from food is preferable, but this should be supplemented when it is inadequate.

While you probably know that dairy products are rich in calcium, you may not be familiar with the wide range of other foods that provide this mineral. Here is a selection of foods that are high in calcium, to help you plan a diet to keep your bones strong.

Food Item	Serving Size	Calcium Content (mg)	Calories
Milk			
Whole	8 oz.	291	150
Skim	8 oz.	302	85
Yogurt (with added milk solids)			
Plain, low-fat	8 oz.	415	145
Fruit, low-fat	8 oz.	343	230
Frozen, fruit	8 oz.	240	223
Frozen, chocolate	8 oz.	160	220
Cheese			
Mozzarella, part skim	1 oz.	207	80
Muenster	1 oz.	203	105
Cheddar	1 oz.	204	115
Ricotta, part skim	4 oz.	335	190
Cottage, low-fat (2%)	4 oz.	78	103
Ice cream, vanilla (11% fat)			
Hard	1 cup	176	270
Soft serve	1 cup	236	375
Ice milk, vanilla			
Hard (4% fat)	1 cup	176	185
Soft serve (3% fat)	1 cup	274	225
Fish and Shellfish			
Oysters (13–19 med.)	1 cup	226	160
Sardines, canned in oil, drained, including bones	3 oz.	372	175
Salmon, pink, canned, including bones	3 oz.	167	120
Shrimp, canned, drained	3 oz.	98	100
Vegetables			
Bok choy, raw	1 cup	74	9

Food Item	Serving Size	Calcium Content (mg)	Calories
Broccoli, cooked, drained, from raw	1 cup	136	40
Broccoli, cooked, drained, from frozen	1 cup	100	50
Soybeans, cooked, drained, from raw	1 cup	131	235
Collards, cooked, drained, from raw	1 cup	357	65
Turnip greens, cooked, drained, from raw (leaves and stems)	1 cup	252	30
Tofu (calcium content may vary depending on processing methods)	4 oz.	108	85
Almonds	1 oz.	75	165

Source: The National Osteoporosis Foundation, *Boning Up on Osteoporosis, A Guide to Prevention and Treatment*, 1991. Reprinted with permission.

PROBLEMS WITH DAIRY PRODUCTS

▶ ▶ ▶ ▶ ▶ ▶ ▶ ▶ ▶ ▶

Dairy products are particularly high in calcium. Skim milk, low-fat milk, yogurt, and low-fat cheeses are excellent sources for gaining calcium and aiding bone health.

Unfortunately, nothing is simple or right for everyone. There are several reasons why many women avoid dairy foods. One issue is a fear of the fat and calories in dairy products. Vegans (strict vegetarians) choose not to consume any animal-derived substances for ethical and health-related reasons. Some women are concerned about the antibiotics and hormones given to dairy cows and the level of pesticide residues and other environmental contaminants in their feed.

People also give up dairy foods because of adverse physical reactions. Dairy products can increase mucous buildup and aggravate sinus and asthma conditions. Another fairly common problem is lactose intolerance, difficulty digesting dairy foods.

Many adults lack the enzyme lactase, which is needed to break down the milk sugar lactose. Consuming milk products can result in gastrointestinal distress and numerous other symptoms. This problem can be alleviated by adding lactase drops to milk, taking lactase pills, or buying milk pretreated with the enzyme. Yogurt containing live acidophilus cultures can be well tolerated by many people who have adverse reactions to regular milk.

If you choose not to drink milk, there are alternatives: calcium-enriched beverages made from soy, rice, or almonds. These beverages have the texture of milk, a delicious taste, and a high calcium content. They taste great with cereal and can be used in recipes as a milk substitute. You can also get calcium and refreshment from enriched orange juice and other fruit juices.

MAXIMIZING CALCIUM ABSORPTION

▸ ▸ ▸ ▸ ▸ ▸ ▸ ▸ ▸ ▸ ▸

As with other nutrients, it is not only how much calcium you take in that counts, it's how much you *absorb* that counts. Age, diet, hormonal status, presence of disease, and use of drugs can influence calcium absorption. Aging by itself brings a diminished ability to absorb calcium.

Bone stores 99 percent of the body's calcium, while blood stores 1 percent. This is a small but critical margin, 8.5–10.5 mg/dL. If the blood level decreases, the bone begins to leach calcium.

The nutrient that enhances calcium absorption is vitamin D in its activated form. Vitamin D allows the calcium to leave the intestine and enter the bloodstream, where it can aid in building bone.

Vitamin D is naturally formed by the body after about a fifteen-minute exposure to sunlight. People who are homebound or not exposed to sunlight for some other reason may have a vitamin D deficiency. Food sources of vitamin D include egg yolks, saltwater fish, liver, and vitamin D–fortified milk or juice.

The RDA for vitamin D is 400 IU (international units). Unless a doctor has specifically prescribed it, higher supplementation is not recommended since too much vitamin D can lead to excessive calcium in the blood.

Two supplements that can interfere with calcium absorption are iron and magnesium. If your doctor recommends these minerals, you should take them at a different time of day than your calcium.

Caffeine, which is in coffee, nonherbal tea, and cola, can inhibit calcium absorption by accelerating excretion. High levels of protein, sodium, and fiber can also interfere with calcium absorption. However, this does not mean these substances should be eliminated, just consumed in moderation and balanced with calcium-rich foods.

CALCIUM AND OTHER SUPPLEMENTS

▸ ▸ ▸ ▸ ▸ ▸ ▸ ▸ ▸ ▸ ▸

You may need to take a calcium supplement if your doctor recommends it, or if you feel you can't get enough calcium from food. The amount of supplementation you need depends on what you're already getting from dietary sources. The goal is to build up to the optimal daily requirement of 1,000 mg for premenopausal women or those taking estrogen; 1,500 mg for postmenopausal women not taking estrogen.

In choosing a supplement, you need to read the label to determine how much *elemental* calcium is in the product. Calcium supplements come in many forms, the most common of which are calcium carbonate and calcium citrate. Types that are not recommended are bone meal and dolomite.

Following are common calcium supplements and their percentage of elemental calcium.

FORM OF CALCIUM SUPPLEMENT	PERCENT OF ELEMENTAL CALCIUM
Calcium carbonate	40
Calcium phosphate (tribasic)	39
Calcium phosphate (dibasic)	30
Calcium citrate	21
Calcium lactate	13
Calcium gluconate	9

Source: The National Osteoporosis Foundation, *Boning Up on Osteoporosis, A Guide to Prevention and Treatment*, 1991. Reprinted with permission.

Research conducted at the HNRCA at Tufts University found that the body utilizes calcium supplements best when the individual dosage does not exceed 500 mg at a time. It was also found that calcium carbonate, the form in the most popular chewable supplements, is absorbed most effectively when taken with meals.

When choosing a supplement, you can ask your doctor or pharmacist to recommend a product that meets the USP (United States Pharmacopeia) standards, which indicate that the tablet will disintegrate in the stomach and be absorbed. Determine how many tablets you'll need to take to obtain your optimal requirement, considering that 100 percent of the RDA is not enough for most midlife women.

And remember, just because you're taking a supplement doesn't mean you can ignore the need to get calcium in your food. Mother Nature always does it best.

TIME TO START THE 4-WEEK WORKOUT PROGRAM

The goal of the workout program is to establish exercise as a regular, pleasurable part of your life. You'll experience immediate benefits: more energy, increased strength and flexibility, a surge of good spirits. Most importantly, you'll establish the healthy habit of exercise and feel proud of your accomplishment.

You may be wondering, "Why a program? Why don't I just start to exercise?" The multiple emotional and physical stresses women face at midlife create a special need for this program. The program provides an organized plan for incorporating regular sessions of aerobic activity, strength training, and stretching into your week. And it offers suggestions on nutrition, relaxation, and other support for the exercise. The structure of a program directs you to focus on taking care of yourself.

Midlife women are often great caregivers, tending to the needs of children, parents, spouses, friends, bosses, and colleagues. Sometimes all this caregiving and responsibility can leave little time and energy to take care of *you*.

The beginning of the program is a time to shift this emphasis just a little—not to neglect other people—but to make it top priority to take care of yourself. You more than deserve it. And the time spent on yourself will give you a surplus of strength and positive energy to do all the other things you need to do for other people.

The number one reason women give for not exercising is: "I don't have time!"

I do sympathize and I understand how busy and overwhelming life can be. I often feel as if I'm running in ten directions and will never get everything done (don't we all!). But I refuse to accept the no-time-for-exercise excuse from anyone.

When you choose to set exercise as a priority and look at your schedule creatively, you *will* find time. Here are suggestions that might help:

MORNING Set your alarm clock a half-hour to an hour earlier to allow yourself time to exercise first thing in the morning. The increase in energy you'll get from working out will more than compensate for losing a little sleep. You'll feel extra alert and energetic all day.

NOON A few days a week, plan to exercise during your lunch hour. If you join a health club or gym near your workplace, you can take a midday class or use the machines. You can also ride a bike, jog, or walk during your lunchtime. Lunchtime workouts are a wonderful way to beat the mid-afternoon slump and feel focused the rest of the workday.

AFTER WORK For many women, this is a favorite time to exercise. It's a terrific way to shake off the tension of work and gain renewed energy for your evening.

The trick is to exercise *as soon as possible* after work, before you get distracted by reading mail, answering calls, rehashing the day, etc. If you get involved in these details and duties, soon it's dinnertime and then you'll be too full to exercise.

You might drive yourself directly to an exercise class or gym from your workplace. Or change into your gear as soon as you get home and go for it. Think of exercise as your number one priority directly after work. The rest will all be there waiting for you when you're finished.

EVENING If all else fails, you can exercise half an hour after you've had a *light* dinner. You can use an at-home exercise machine (such as a treadmill) while watching TV, do an exercise video, or the 4-Week Workout. If you're really ambitious, you can go to an evening exercise class or check out the nighttime scene at a health club.

If you're the mother of young children it may seem as if you don't have a moment to spare for exercise. But when you're doing the hard work of being a mom, you need to reserve this special time *for* you. Exercise is a must for maintaining your strength and sanity for the juggling act.

As Kathy, a mother of three children, says, "I have to organize my time away from work, kids, and husband to make sure I have time to exercise. It's not easy, but when something is really important to you, you find time to do it." Kathy plans her exercise sessions a month in advance and keeps them as she would any other appointment.

Ultimately, your child will benefit from your taking the time to exercise. You'll have more energy and often be in a better mood. You'll also be a good role model, showing your child that exercise is important. Many of us had mothers who didn't exercise regularly, and this may be one reason why it's so hard to establish it as a habit.

You can open your child up to the joy and pleasure of different forms of exercise. Your child can learn from you that fitness goes way beyond the competitive games of physical education.

Every mother faces a unique set of scheduling challenges. You may be able to pick and choose from the following suggestions on how to find time to exercise.

▸ If you have very young children, nap time can be your time to exercise and rejuvenate yourself.
▸ Take a child/mother exercise class (offered at many Y's, continuing education centers, and health clubs).
▸ Take your child along on fitness walks and bike rides.
▸ Join a health club with baby-sitting services or kids' activities.
▸ When you drop your child off for an activity or class, use the time before pickup to do an exercise session.
▸ Ask your childcare provider to stay an extra hour a few times a week so you can concentrate on working out.
▸ Trade off child-watching with a neighbor to free up exercise time.
▸ Plan physical outings with your kids whenever possible—walking, hiking, biking, swimming.

"If I didn't make an appointment to exercise, I wouldn't do it." This is a comment I hear over and over again from my clients.

It's one of the simplest keys to success in your fitness program: *Make an appointment to exercise.* I have had hundreds of women tell me this method works.

When you vaguely decide you'll exercise sometime later in the day, the day flies by and often you don't exercise. If you set a firm appointment for a fixed time, you will.

You can establish this healthy habit during the 4-Week Workout Program. Every Sunday, consult your datebook or calendar and write down your fitness appointments for the week. Write them in ink!

Consider these appointments as mandatory as any others on your calendar and make a firm commitment to keep them. Imagine I'm going to show up at your door for a personal training session, raring to go, at the appointed time.

The hour at which you schedule your appointments is a personal choice. The best time to exercise is the time you'll do it. You may be a bright-eyed morning person, or it may take Arnold Schwarzenegger to drag you out of bed for a workout. You may be able to schedule a session at lunchtime, or you may prefer to wait until the evening when all your duties are done. There's no optimal time to exercise, except the time that's best for you.

Consider your energy level and your lifestyle when planning your exercise sessions. If you're not sure, set appointments at various times and see what works for you.

The amount of time you'll need to schedule depends on which form of exercise you'll do that day. If you're planning to do the Strength Training Routine, give yourself about half an hour.

The time needed for aerobic activities depends on the form of the activities. After you decide on your activities, you can consult the charts in Chapter 8 for the length of the session recommended for your fitness level. Add time to change clothes, travel to the activity (if necessary), and about ten minutes for the Flexibility Cooldown.

The first appointment to schedule is the most important: your date to start the 4-Week Workout Program. Set yourself a deadline no later than two weeks from now. You want to keep rolling while you're inspired.

Since the program is not very time-consuming, it can be done during any normal month when you're working and following your usual schedule. Try to choose a block of time when there won't be any major disruptions or unusual demands on your time. Expect to spend three to four hours a week on all the elements of the program.

The basic elements of the program are:

- Three sessions of aerobic activity each week
- Two sessions of the Strength Training Routine for strength training and flexibility
- The Lifestyle Lifts

Once you've got your starting date, mark it boldly on your calendar and do your absolute best to keep the date. But if for some reason you can't, start as soon as possible. Don't let any setbacks keep you stuck in a rut. Plunge in and you'll reap the rewards.

Here is a sample exercise calendar for the four weeks of the program. Debbie, a forty-nine-year-old woman, has determined that she is Fitness Level 2, according to the tests and criteria. Her calendar will show you the basic ingredients of the 4-Week Workout Program. How you select and schedule your own activities is up to you.

	SUNDAY	MONDAY	TUESDAY	WEDNESDAY	THURSDAY	FRIDAY	SATURDAY
WEEK 1		1 25-min. walk Review Calcium Intake	2 Strength Training Routine Start drinking more water!	3 25-min. walk	4 Strength Training Routine Posture check	5	6 25-min. walk Buy calcium supplements
WEEK 2	7 25-min. walk with Arlene	8 Strength Training Routine Practice deep breathing	9 Go to health food store for healthy snacks	10 Strength Training Routine	11	12 30-min. walk Practice deep breathing	13 Gym day! 15-min. swim 15-min. bike
WEEK 3	14 Hike and picnic with David—bring the water bottle!	15	16 30-min. walk Strength Training Routine	17 Low-fat cooking class at the Y	18 20-min. bike Strength Training Routine	19	20 Shopping day, buy new leggings
WEEK 4	21	22 Try step class at gym (Eat small frequent meals this week)	23	24 Strength Training Routine (Pay attention to form and breathing)	25 15-min. swim Herbal facial at home Practice progressive relaxation	26 20-min. walk Strength Training Routine	27 45-min. walk with Arlene 5 p.m. massage
	28	29	30				

1. HAVE A COMPLETE CHECKUP WITH A PHYSICIAN

Before embarking on a new exercise program, it's recommended that you have a complete physical examination with a physician, including a stress test, blood workup, and bone density test.

Review your test results with your physician to see if there are any conditions or weaknesses which will affect your exercise capabilities. Discuss which forms of exercise are appropriate for you in the case of physical limitations. Explain to your doctor what you are planning to do in the Workout Program and get his or her approval. If it's considered necessary, schedule office visits to monitor your reaction during the four weeks of the program.

2. FIND YOUR FITNESS LEVEL AND PLAN YOUR AEROBIC ACTIVITIES

Before starting the Workout Program, refer to the Fitness Level Test and criteria in Chapter 6 to determine your level. Then you can check the Aerobic Charts at the end of Chapter 8 to see which activities are appropriate for you.

You'll be doing aerobics at least three times a week. Choose two to five activities to try during the month of the program. At least one should be an indoor activity that is not dependent on the weather.

Once you select your activities, create a list of what you need to prepare for each one. This may include buying gear, finding an appropriate place for the workout, joining a class or a club. Then you can take care of these steps so you're ready to go by your program starting date.

3. GET YOUR GEAR

The primary gear you'll need is a pair of quality exercise sneakers. Don't plan to wear a pair of old tennis sneakers for the Workout Program—you need serious support. It's well worth investing in a pair of good sneakers that will reduce the risk of injury and make your exercising life much easier.

When you first shop for sneakers, it may seem as if there's a type for everything but dishwashing. Don't be overwhelmed by the choices; visit a store with knowledgeable salespeople who will take the time to help. If you're planning to do several forms of aerobics, a good cross-training sneaker is your best bet, unless you have the closet space for a whole sneaker wardrobe. If you're planning to walk or jog as your main activity, select a running sneaker.

Your workout clothes depend on the activity and your own personal style. Some women love to layer old T-shirts, leggings, and sweatshirts, while others feel great in shiny, sleek leotards. The only rules are that your workout clothes should provide full range of motion and be appealing to you. Have a mini-wardrobe of exercise outfits you look forward to putting on.

I strongly recommend wearing a sports bra during workouts.

You'll be more comfortable with support and your breasts will thank you.

For cold-weather workouts, wear layers of loose clothing, with a first layer, closest to the body, that absorbs the sweat. Cover your head and ears and wear warm socks. (I'm starting to sound like a mother, but it's very important!)

The other gear you need for aerobic workouts will depend on the activity—it may be a set of steps, a tennis racquet, or a tuned-up bike. Get whatever you need beforehand so you're ready to rock the first week of the program.

To prepare for the Strength Training Routine, identify a place in your home where you have sufficient room to stand, stretch, lie down, and lean against a wall and a chair or sofa. If the room has a foam-backed carpet, you can use a towel or sheet for the lying-down exercises. If not, you can purchase a portable exercise mat at a sporting goods store.

For the Strength Training Routine you'll also need hand and ankle weights, which are also available at sporting goods stores. The size of the weights depends on your fitness level.

LEVEL 1	3-lb. hand weights No ankle weights
LEVEL 2	5-lb. hand weights 3-lb. ankle weights
LEVEL 3	8-lb. hand weights 5 lb. ankle weights
WOMEN WITH OSTEOPOROSIS	1- to 3-lb. hand weights 1- to 3-lb. ankle weights

4. TELL YOUR FRIENDS AND FAMILY It's helpful to tell your close friends and family you're embarking on the Workout Program and explain your goals to them. Let them know that you're serious about the program and it means a lot to you. Tell them you'd appreciate their support and understanding if your schedule is a little different than usual.

Regardless of your partner's reaction to the Workout Program, carry on with your plan. The bottom line is that the program is an effort you're making for your own well-being.

If one of your friends expresses a lot of interest in the program, see if she wants to be your workout buddy. It's very supportive to have a buddy, providing she's disciplined and committed to the program. She can help you get back on track if you start to miss exercise appointments.

On the other hand, if your buddy cancels the exercise dates, it can be all too easy for you to follow. Talk it out beforehand to be sure she really intends to go through with the exercise plan. If she's not certain, you can start by scheduling a few of your exercise sessions together and see how it goes.

IMPORTANT NOTE: The following four chapters provide guidelines and workouts that are appropriate for women in Fitness Levels 1–3. However, if you have been diagnosed as having osteoporosis, regardless of your fitness level, there is a special program and workout for you in Chapter 17. Please refer to this chapter for your program.

CHECKLIST TO GET READY FOR THE PROGRAM
▶ ▶ ▶ ▶ ▶ ▶ ▶ ▶ ▶ ▶ ▶

1. Have a medical examination and get your doctor's go-ahead.
2. Set a starting date and write it down in your calendar or datebook.
3. Plan the aerobic activities you want to do. Sign up for classes or join a health club if you wish.
4. Obtain quality sneakers, comfortable workout clothes, weights, and any other equipment you need for your aerobic activities.
5. Identify a good space to do the Strength Training Routine.
6. Tell your friends and family what you plan to do. If you have a friend who'd like to participate, show her this book.
7. Make a firm commitment to stay with the Workout Program and consider exercise a top priority.

WEEK 1 OF THE 4-WEEK WORKOUT PROGRAM

This week you will experience for yourself the power and pleasure of a balanced, challenging exercise program.

The first step is to look at your datebook or calendar and decide on the best time to exercise. Then *write down your exercise appointments for Week 1*. You should schedule two sessions of the Strength Training Routine and three sessions of Aerobic Activity. These can be scheduled on alternating days, or you can do the Strength Training Routine and an aerobic session on the same day. If you're accustomed to exercise, you always have the option of scheduling additional days of aerobics or sports.

For this first week of the program, try to select an Aerobic Activity with which you're familiar. If you've been sedentary, walking is a safe choice. Check the charts at the end of Chapter 8 to determine whether this activity is suitable for your Fitness Level. (If you haven't determined your Fitness Level according to the criteria in Chapter 6, please do so before continuing.)

The aerobic charts will give you guidelines on the type, duration, and intensity of the aerobic activity you choose. If you find it too complicated to measure intensity by your heart rate this week, take it slow and use your common sense instead. You should be able to speak while exercising, and slow down the pace if you feel your heart pounding or if you experience shortness of breath.

You can be flexible with the duration of your aerobic sessions this week if you're out of practice. If you're a beginner, you may need to "bank" your time: Do ten minutes of aerobics, rest, and do ten minutes later in the day. How long you wait in between segments depends on how you feel.

The first week is not a good time to push yourself, except maybe to push yourself to get up and do it. Set a manageable goal: to put on your sneakers and do an aerobic activity three times a week. If you keep your exercise appointments you're already on your way to seeing and feeling results.

The other goal this week and throughout the program is to do the Strength Training Routine twice a week. Before starting, be sure you have:

▸ Hand and ankle weights that are suitable for your Fitness Level (according to the chart in Chapter 12)
▸ Sneakers and comfortable workout clothes
▸ A mat or carpet
▸ Adequate space with a chair or sofa nearby

Read through the instructions and look at the photographs once or twice to familiarize yourself with the exercises. You'll notice that there are different models demonstrating each week's exercises. You may be interested to know that none of the midlife women in the photographs is a professional model; they are clients, colleagues, and relatives who stay in great shape by working out. These "real-life" women manage to exercise regularly while they juggle busy professional and personal lives — what an inspiration!

After you've reviewed the exercises, put on some of your favorite music. Turn off the phone and pretend your personal trainer is there with you, ready to lead you through a special workout. Let's begin.

WARM-UP

FOR HEAD AND SHOULDERS

STARTING POSITION Stand with your legs slightly apart, knees soft. Check your posture: shoulders should be relaxed, spine long, weight to your heels. Breathe deeply into your abdomen.

ACTION Inhale and bring your arms up to your sides and overhead. Exhale and soften your knees as you bring your arms down. Repeat eight times, up and down.

Tilt your head to the right side, down to center, and left. Reverse, making three slow half circles to each side.

Roll your right shoulder back; left shoulder back, four times. Turn your toes out slightly and shift your weight to the right and left (a lunge) as you're rolling your shoulders. Repeat eight times.

FOR UPPER BACK

STARTING POSITION	Stand tall with your legs hip-width apart.
ACTION	Lift your arms to the sides. Bend your knees and bring your arms and upper back forward as if you're hugging a big beach ball. Inhale and open your arms out to the sides as you straighten your legs. Repeat four times.

Place your hands on top of your thighs and bend your knees, turn your toes out slightly, and bend your torso forward. Reach your right shoulder forward and look up to the left. Hold ten seconds and breathe. Switch to the other side and hold ten seconds. Repeat four times on each side.

Keep your knees bent and toes forward. Inhale and curl your tailbone under. Exhale and extend your tailbone toward the ceiling. Repeat three times. Keep your knees bent and slowly roll up.

FOR FULL BODY

STARTING POSITION	Stand tall.
ACTION	Walk in place. Punch your arms forward, to the sides, and overhead, eight times in each direction. Do two times through.

STRENGTH EXERCISES

NOTE: The starting position and action for all three levels are the same on the following muscle-strength-building exercises. The repetitions in the initial *Action* section are for Level 1. However, additional sets, repetitions, and/or weights are given for Levels 2 and 3. Women with low bone density/osteoporosis, please refer to the strength workout in Chapter 17.

ONE-ARM ROW

▸ ▸ ▸ ▸ ▸ ▸ ▸ ▸ ▸ ▸ ▸ ▸ ▸ ▸ ▸ ▸

Benefits rhomboids (mid-back), latissimus dorsi (back), biceps (front of arms)

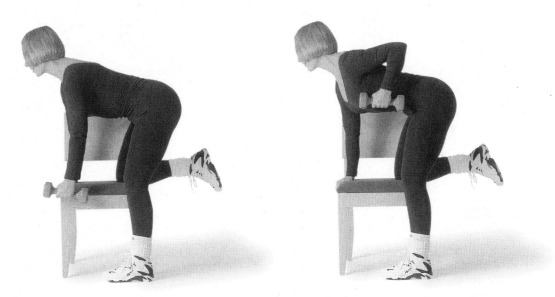

STARTING POSITION Stand beside a couch or chair. Rest your right knee and hand on it. Back is parallel to the floor, head down. Hold your 3-lb. weight in your left hand, extending your left arm down.

ACTION Exhale and bend your left elbow, bringing your arm up so your elbow is above your back. Inhale as you bring your arm down. Pull up and release down eight times with the left arm; then switch sides and do eight times with the right.

HELPFUL HINT Use your back muscles for the lift (your shoulder blade should move with the action).

LEVEL 2 Do two sets of eight on each side using 5-lb. weights.

LEVEL 3 Do two sets of ten on each side using 8-lb. weights.

Benefits quadriceps (front of thighs)

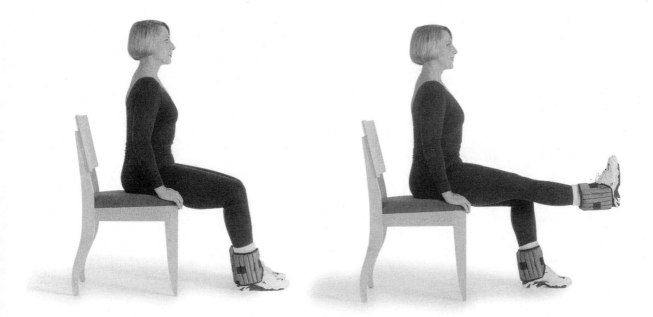

STARTING POSITION	Sit on the edge of your couch or chair, keeping your spine long, feet flat on the floor.
ACTION	Exhale and extend your right leg; inhale and bring your leg down. Repeat eight times on each side.
HELPFUL HINT	Keep your torso upright (you can support yourself with your hands on the couch or chair).
LEVEL 2	Do two sets of eight on each side, wearing 3-lb. ankle weights.
LEVEL 3	Do two sets of ten on each side, wearing 5-lb. ankle weights.

Benefits forearms and wrists

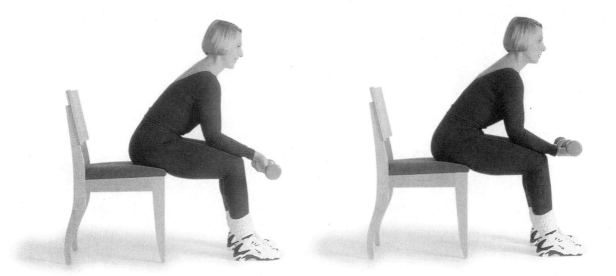

STARTING POSITION	Sit on the edge of a couch or chair, feet flat on the floor. Rest your forearms on top of your thighs, palms up, holding 3-lb. weights.
ACTION	Exhale and curl your wrists in; inhale, extend out. Repeat eight times.
LEVEL 2	Do two sets of eight, using 5-lb. weights.
LEVEL 3	Do two sets of ten, using 5-lb. weights.

Benefits forearms and wrists

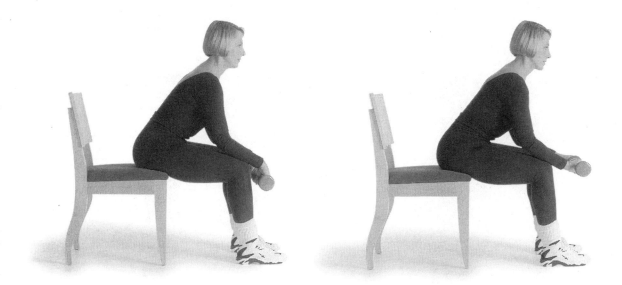

STARTING POSITION Sit on the edge of a couch or chair, feet flat on the floor. Rest your forearms on top of your thighs, palms down, holding 3-lb. weights.

ACTION Exhale and curl your wrists up; inhale, lower down. Repeat eight times.

LEVEL 2 Do two sets of eight, using 5-lb. weights.

LEVEL 3 Do two sets of ten, using 5-lb. weights.

LEG CURLS

▸ ▸

Benefits hamstrings (back of thighs)

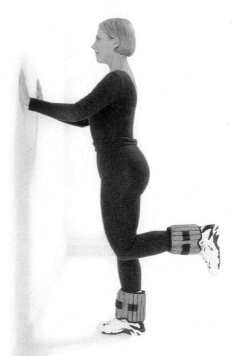

STARTING POSITION	Stand with both legs hip-width apart and place both hands against the wall for balance.
ACTION	Exhale and bend at the knee, bringing your left heel up to your buttocks. Inhale while slowly releasing down. Repeat eight times on each side.
HELPFUL HINTS	Keep your abdomen firm to avoid arching your lower back, and keep your knees together.
LEVEL 2	Two sets of eight on each side, wearing 3-lb. ankle weights.
LEVEL 3	Two sets of ten on each side, wearing 5-lb. ankle weights.

▸ ▸

Benefits pectorals (chest), triceps (back of arms)

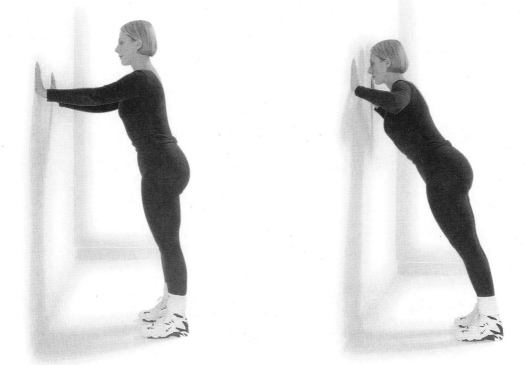

STARTING POSITION	Standing, place both hands on the wall, fingertips facing up.
ACTION	Inhale and bend your elbows as you lean into the wall. Exhale and push out, so your arms straighten. Do eight wall pushups.
LEVEL 2	Do two sets of eight wall pushups.

Level 3, Modified Pushup, continued on page 96

Benefits pectorals (chest), triceps (back of arms)

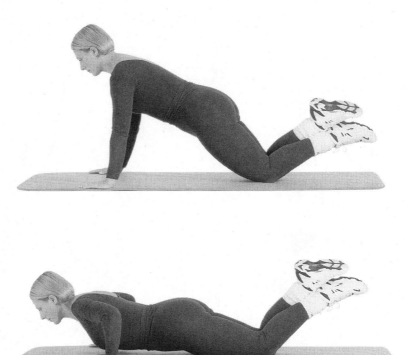

STARTING POSITION   Start on your hands and knees facedown, with ankles crossed and arms straight.

ACTION   Inhale and bend your elbows as you lower yourself almost to the floor. Exhale and push up until your arms are straight. Do two sets of ten.

WING-OUT

▸ ▸

Benefits rotator cuff (shoulder joint) and posterior deltoid (back of shoulder)

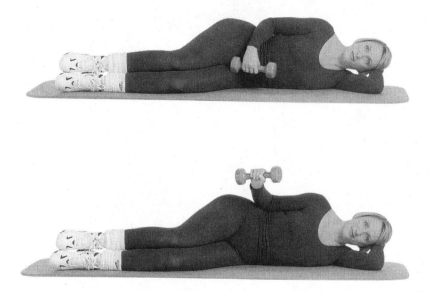

STARTING POSITION Lie on your left side with both knees bent, right elbow resting on your hip. Hold your 3-lb. weight in your right hand, in front of your navel, palm down.

ACTION Keeping your elbow touching your side, exhale and lift the weight toward ceiling, inhale and lower down to navel. Repeat ten times on each side.

LEVEL 2 Do two sets of eight, using 3-lb. weights.

LEVEL 3 Do two sets of ten, using 5-lb. weights.

Benefits abdominals and sphincter muscles

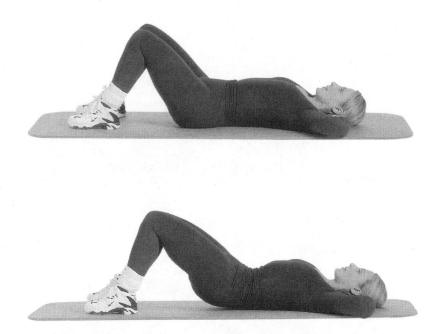

STARTING POSITION	Lie on your back with your knees bent and feet flat on the floor.
ACTION	Inhale, filling up your abdomen. Exhale and gently push your lower back into the floor while tightening your sphincter muscles. Hold for three seconds, then release. Repeat ten times.
HELPFUL HINT	As you exhale, your lower back will flatten into the floor.
LEVEL 2	Same.
LEVEL 3	Same.

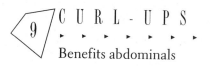
Benefits abdominals

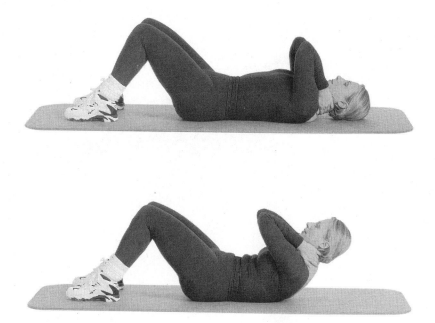

STARTING POSITION	Lie on your back with your knees bent, feet flat on the floor. Clasp both hands behind your neck and bring your elbows forward.
ACTION	Exhale as you tilt your pelvis and lift your upper back off the floor. Inhale as you slowly release down. Repeat eight times.
HELPFUL HINTS	Keep your chin off your chest and keep your neck as relaxed as possible.

Levels 2 and 3, Curl-Ups, continued on page 100

Benefits abdominals

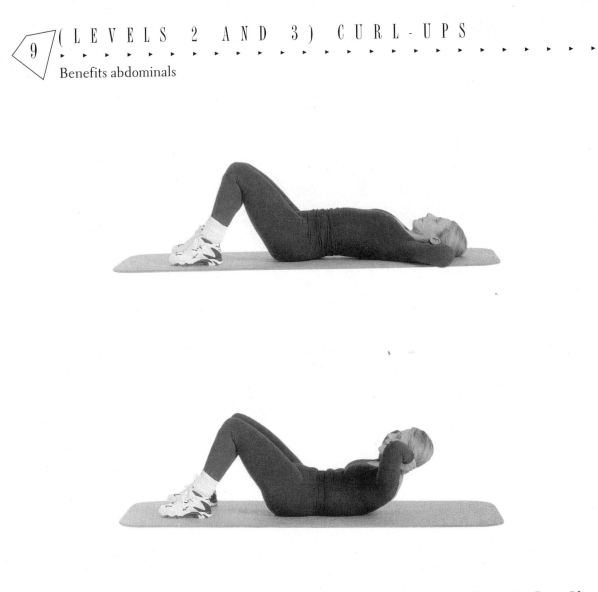

STARTING POSITION Lie on your back with your knees bent, feet flat on the floor. Clasp both hands behind your head and bring your elbows out to the side.

ACTION Exhale as you tilt your pelvis and lift your upper back off the floor. Inhale as you slowly release down.

LEVEL 2 Do two sets of eight.

LEVEL 3 Do two sets of ten.

Benefits abdominals

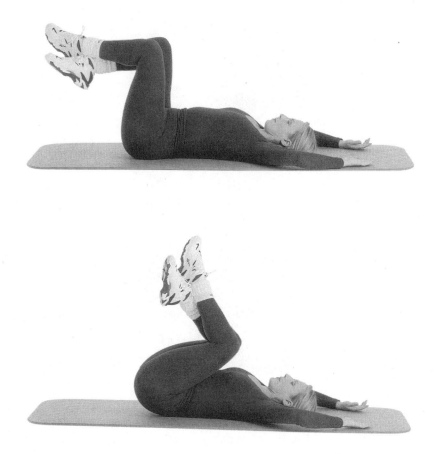

STARTING POSITION	Lie on your back with your knees bent, arms overhead on the floor. Lift your feet off the floor, bringing your knees in to your chest, and cross your ankles.
ACTION	Exhale and lift your lower back off the ground, curling in. Inhale as you release. Repeat eight times.
HELPFUL HINT	Do this exercise slowly, as a small movement.
LEVEL 2	Do two sets of eight.
LEVEL 3	Do two sets of ten.

‣ ‣ ‣ ‣ ‣ ‣ ‣ ‣ ‣ ‣ ‣ ‣ ‣ ‣ ‣ ‣ ‣ ‣ ‣ ‣

Benefits abdominals and obliques (waist)

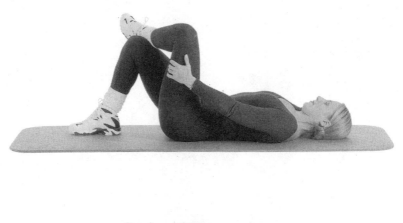

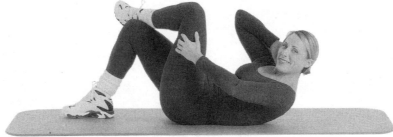

STARTING POSITION Lie on your back with both knees bent. Cross your left foot over your right knee, letting the left knee turn out. Place your right hand behind your head and left arm holding onto the outside of your left thigh.

ACTION Exhale as you lift yourself toward your left knee. Inhale as you slowly lower. Repeat eight times on each side.

LEVEL 2 Do two sets of eight on each side.

LEVEL 3 Do two sets of ten on each side.

Benefits erector spinae (muscles on both sides of spine) and lower back

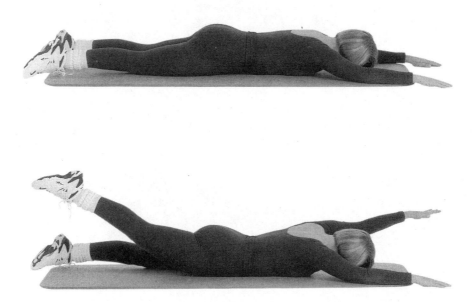

STARTING POSITION	Lie on your stomach, facedown, and extend both arms overhead on the floor.
ACTION	Keeping your limbs straight, exhale as you lift your left arm and right leg. Head remains facing down as you hold for three counts, then lower. Repeat ten times, alternating sides.
HELPFUL HINT	Think of Superman as you lift up.
LEVEL 2	Same.
LEVEL 3	Same.

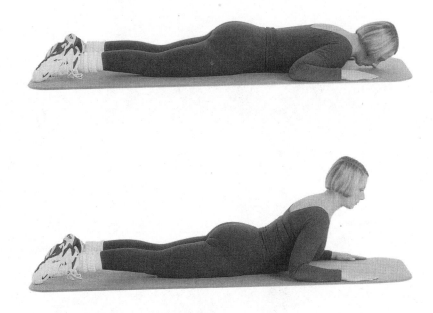

STARTING POSITION	Lie on your stomach with your hands by your head, elbows bent at right angles and forearms on the floor, facedown.
ACTION	Exhale as you press your hands into the floor and raise your chest until you're arching slightly. Hold for three counts, then inhale as you release down. Repeat eight times.
HELPFUL HINTS	Keep your pelvis on the floor and look down while pushing up.
LEVEL 2	Do eight press-ups.
LEVEL 3	Do ten press-ups.

Benefits erector spinae and latissimus dorsi (back)

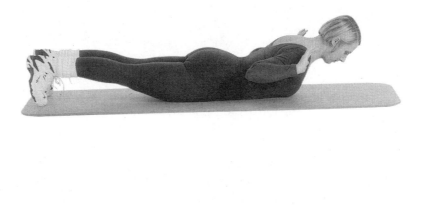

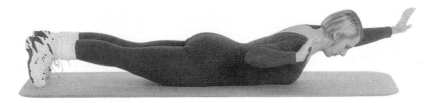

STARTING POSITION	Lie on your stomach with your hands by your head, elbows bent at right angles and forearms on the floor, head down. Push onto the balls of your feet so both knees are off the floor. Press your shoulder blades together and lift your arms off the floor.
ACTION	Alternate, first pushing your left arm and then your right straight in front of your head. Repeat five times, alternating arms.
HELPFUL HINT	Breathe naturally throughout the exercise.
LEVEL 2	Do eight pushes with each arm, alternating.
LEVEL 3	Do ten pushes with each arm, alternating.

Hold each stretch for ten to thirty seconds.

QUADRICEP STRETCH   Lie on your stomach, face down. Bend your right knee behind you and grab hold of your foot. Bring your heel toward your buttocks, as close as possible without straining, while breathing deeply. Slowly release down. Repeat with left leg.

BACK STRETCH   Lie on your stomach, facedown. Use your hands to press up and back onto your heels while bending your knees. Stretch your arms and fingers in front of you on the floor, stretching out your back.

HAMSTRING STRETCH   Turn onto your back. Bend both knees and place your feet flat on the floor. Bend your right knee in to your chest, then extend the leg straight up, keeping both hips on the floor. If you want additional stretch, you can wrap both hands around your thigh and gently pull the leg in toward your body. Release by bending your knee, then lowering it to floor. Repeat with left leg.

CHEST STRETCH   Roll onto one side, then use your hands to help yourself up to standing. Go into a doorway and hold on to the sides with your elbows bent at 90-degree angles. Step forward with one leg, as if you're walking into the room, so that your elbows are slightly behind you and your chest is open.

NECK AND SHOULDER STRETCH   Stand tall, then tilt your head to the left side and the right. Extend your right arm up and stretch; then stretch your left arm. Roll your shoulders back a few times. Shake out any spots that feel tight.

L I F E S T Y L E   L I F T S

INCREASE YOUR CALCIUM INTAKE   Begin by reviewing your present calcium intake. Check the chart of calcium-rich foods in Chapter 11 and write down the amount of these foods and beverages you consume in an average week. Then add up your total and divide by seven. Compare this number with the optimal amount:

- 1,000 mg for premenopausal women or those taking estrogen
- 1,500 mg for menopausal or postmenopausal women not taking estrogen.

    If your daily calcium intake is lower than this recommended amount, first check with your physician to ensure you don't have any conditions which contraindicate supplementation. Then you can plan how to boost your daily intake of this bone-building nutrient.

The best way to gain calcium is the natural way — through nutritious foods and drinks. You can also add a high-quality calcium supplement to your daily routine. Remember, you need 400 IU of vitamin D each day to facilitate calcium absorption.

DRINK MORE WATER　One of the best things you can do for yourself is also one of the easiest: Drink lots of water!

Among other benefits, water will help cleanse your body, make you less likely to overeat, improve your skin tone, maintain your hydration level, and help prevent constipation. Drinking six to eight glasses of pure water a day will deliver these benefits.

It might help to write down how much water you're drinking each day until six to eight glasses becomes a regular habit. You can also get a handy sports water bottle to refill and keep nearby.

PAY ATTENTION TO YOUR POSTURE　In the midlife years, posture is not only a cosmetic concern, it's a health issue. Good posture, along with balanced exercise and nutrition, helps to prevent fractures and back or neck pain.

No one expects you to change a lifetime of habits in the first week of this program. But you can start to pay attention to your posture and notice what you'd like to improve. Slight inward curves at the neck and lower back and a gentle outward curve at the upper back indicate good alignment.

Here are ways you can improve your posture and alignment:

- ‣ Practice standing up tall with your weight balanced on both legs.
- ‣ When you sit or stand, bring your shoulders down and back.
- ‣ Carry your pocketbook or bags on alternating sides to cultivate balanced muscles. Try a backpack as an option.
- ‣ Wear low or moderate heels to avoid shortened leg muscles and lower back compression.
- ‣ Work in a well-designed chair that allows you to keep your feet flat on the floor and your knees level with or slightly higher than your hips.
- ‣ Try not to sit with your legs crossed for a long period of time without shifting.
- ‣ Position your computer screen and television set so you can view them without looking down. Bring reading material up to eye level.
- ‣ Hold the phone up to your ear; don't jam it between your head and shoulder. Consider getting a lightweight headset if you're on

the phone a lot. (You can use a speakerphone, if you don't mind sounding like you're under water.)

- ▸ Bend from the knees, not the waist, whenever you lift something. Carry heavy items in both arms, close to your body.
- ▸ Staying in one position is not natural, even with good posture. Be kinetic: stretch, shift positions, and walk around as much as possible.

CHECKLIST FOR WEEK 1

1. Write down your exercise appointments: three sessions of Aerobic Activity and two sessions of the Strength Training Routine.
2. Do an Aerobic Activity at least three times this week, for the duration recommended in the chart for your fitness level. Don't forget the Warm-up and Cooldown.
3. Do the Strength Training Routine twice this week.
4. Review your calcium intake and increase it to the optimal amount if necessary.
5. Drink six to eight glasses of water each day.
6. Evaluate your posture and identify areas you'd like to improve.
7. Pat yourself on the back. Getting started on an exercise program can be the hardest part!

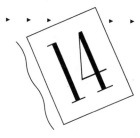

WEEK 2 OF THE 4-WEEK WORKOUT PROGRAM

The first step of Week 2 of the program is to write down your exercise appointments: three sessions of Aerobic Activity and two of the Strength Training Routine. You can do the same type of aerobics you did last week for two of the days, and a new activity for the third workout if you're feeling adventurous.

The aerobic charts will recommend the duration of the type of exercise you choose. For intensity, you can refer to the Borg RPE Scale in Chapter 6 to measure your rate of perceived exertion. Check to see if the RPE is appropriate for your fitness level, and adjust your intensity if needed. Don't forget to warm up and cool down before and after aerobics.

This week you'll continue to build muscle strength and flexibility with the second Strength Training Routine. In this workout and in weeks 3 and 4, the Warm-up and Flexibility Cooldown sequences are the same as in Week 1, while the strength exercises vary.

When you're ready to work out, put on some music that gets you going and have fun!

W A R M - U P

▸ ▸

FOR HEAD AND SHOULDERS
▸ ▸ ▸ ▸ ▸ ▸ ▸ ▸ ▸ ▸

STARTING POSITION Stand with your legs slightly apart, knees soft. Check your posture: shoulders should be relaxed, spine long, weight to your heels. Breathe deeply into your abdomen.

ACTION Inhale and bring your arms up to your sides and overhead. Exhale and soften your knees as you bring your arms down. Repeat eight times, up and down.

Tilt your head to the right side, down to center, and left. Reverse, making three slow half-circles to each side.

Roll your right shoulder back, then your left shoulder back, four times. Add a lunge, right side and left side, as you're rolling your shoulders. Repeat eight times.

FOR UPPER BACK
▸ ▸ ▸ ▸ ▸ ▸ ▸ ▸ ▸ ▸

STARTING POSITION Stand tall with your legs hip-width apart.

ACTION Lift your arms to the sides. Bend your knees and bring your arms and upper back forward as if you're hugging a big beach ball. Inhale and open your arms out to the sides as you straighten your legs. Repeat four times.

Place your hands on top of your thighs and bend your knees, turn your toes out slightly and bend your torso forward. Reach your right shoulder forward and look up to the left. Hold ten seconds and breathe. Switch to the other side and hold ten seconds. Repeat four times on each side.

Keep your knees bent and toes forward. Inhale and curl your tailbone under. Exhale and extend your tailbone toward the ceiling. Repeat three times. Keeping your knees bent, slowly roll up.

FOR FULL BODY
▸ ▸ ▸ ▸ ▸ ▸ ▸ ▸ ▸ ▸

STARTING POSITION Stand tall.

ACTION Walk in place. Punch your arms forward, to the sides, and overhead, eight times in each direction. Do two times through.

STRENGTH EXERCISES

▸   ▸

NOTE: The starting position and action for all three levels are the same on the following muscle-strength-building exercises. The repetitions in the initial *Action* section are for Level 1. However, additional sets, repetitions, and/or weights are given for Levels 2 and 3. Women with low bone density/osteoporosis, please refer to the strength workout in Chapter 17.

1 CHEST PRESS

▸   ▸

Benefits pectorals (chest)

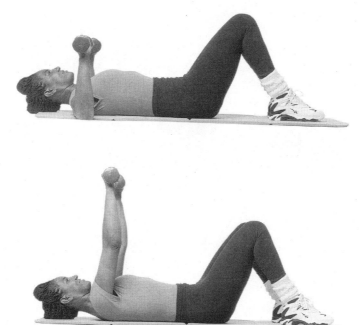

STARTING POSITION	Lie on your back on the mat with both knees bent and feet flat on the floor. With your arms out to the sides and elbows bent, hold 3-lb. weights with your palms forward, forearms off the floor.
ACTION	Exhale and extend your arms straight out over your chest, straightening the elbows. Inhale and return to starting position. Repeat eight times.
LEVEL 2	Do two sets of eight, using 5-lb. weights.
LEVEL 3	Do two sets of ten, using 8-lb. weights.

Benefits gluteus medius and maximus (buttocks), abductors (outer thighs)

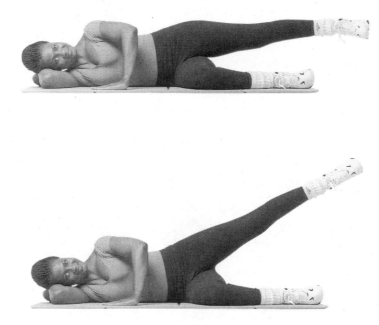

STARTING POSITION Lie on your right side with your right knee bent and left leg extended, head relaxed on your arm. Rest your left hand about six inches in front of your body for balance.

ACTION Exhale as you lift your left leg. Inhale as you lower your leg down. Do two sets of eight, then repeat on the other side.

HELPFUL HINTS Keep both hips facing forward, and top leg parallel to the floor. Leg should not go higher than a 45-degree angle from the floor.

LEVEL 2 Use 3-lb. ankle weights on ankles or above your knee. Do two sets of eight.

LEVEL 3 Use 5-lb. ankle weights on ankles or above your knee. Do two sets of ten.

Benefits adductors (inner thighs)

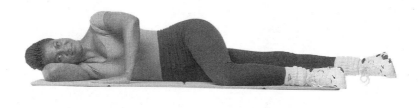

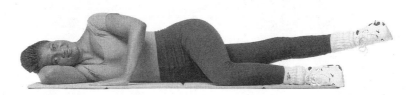

STARTING POSITION Lie on your right side with your right leg straight, left knee bent and resting on the floor in front of you, head relaxed on your arm. Rest your left hand about six inches from your chest for balance.

ACTION Exhale as you lift your right leg. Inhale as you lower your leg. Do two sets of eight, then repeat on the other side.

LEVEL 2 Use 3-lb. weights on ankles or above the knee. Do two sets of eight.

LEVEL 3 Use 5-lb. weights on ankles or above the knee. Do two sets of ten.

Benefits biceps (front of arms)

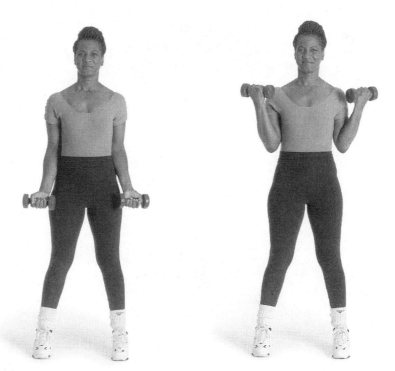

STARTING POSITION	Stand with your legs hip-width apart, knees slightly bent. Hold 3-lb. weights with palms facing forward, elbows at sides.
ACTION	Exhale and bend both elbows, bringing weights up to shoulders. Inhale and slowly release down. Repeat eight times.
HELPFUL HINT	Elbows remain at sides.
LEVEL 2	Do two sets of eight, using 5-lb. weights.
LEVEL 3	Do two sets of ten, using 8-lb. weights.

Benefits deltoids (shoulders)

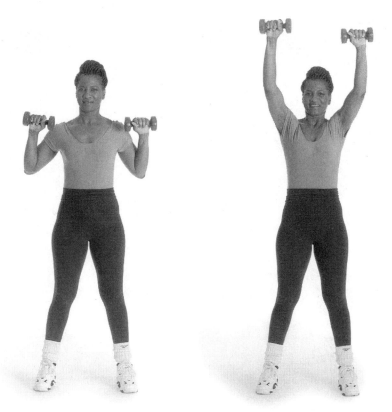

STARTING POSITION	Stand with your legs hip-width apart and knees slightly bent. Hold 3-lb. weights by your shoulders, with palms facing forward.
ACTION	Exhale and slowly extend your arms straight overhead. Inhale and bend elbows as you lower weights to shoulders. Repeat eight times.
	Keep your torso still, firm, and lifted during presses to avoid back discomfort.
HELPFUL HINT	Do two sets of eight, using 5-lb. weights.
LEVEL 2	Do two sets of ten, using 8-lb. weights.
LEVEL 3	

Benefits triceps (back of arms)

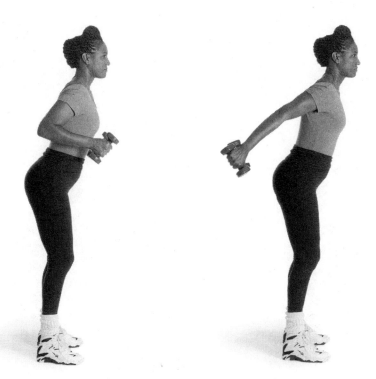

STARTING POSITION   Stand with your legs hip-width apart, knees slightly bent. Hold 3-lb. weights with palms facing each other, elbows bent and slightly behind you.

ACTION   Exhale and straighten arms back. Inhale and bend arms back to starting position. Repeat eight times.

HELPFUL HINT   Upper arms remain stationary.

LEVEL 2   Do two sets of eight, using 5-lb. weights.

LEVEL 3   Do two sets of ten, using 8-lb. weights.

Benefits abdominals and sphincter muscles

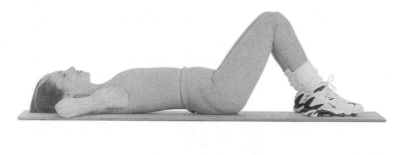

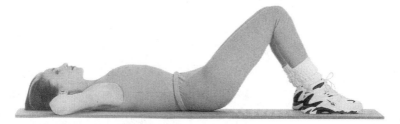

STARTING POSITION	Lie on your back with your knees bent and feet flat on the floor.
ACTION	Inhale, filling up your abdomen. Exhale and gently push your lower back into the floor while tightening your sphincter muscles. Hold for three seconds, then release. Repeat ten times.
HELPFUL HINT	As you exhale, your abdominals will flatten into the floor.
LEVEL 2	Same.
LEVEL 3	Same.

▶ ▶

Benefits abdominals

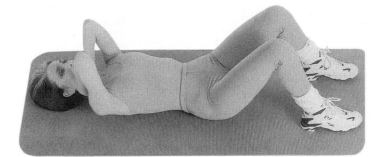

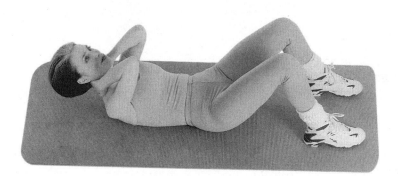

STARTING POSITION	Lie on your back with your knees bent, feet flat on the floor. Clasp both hands behind your neck and bring your elbows forward.
ACTION	Exhale as you tilt your pelvis, then lift your upper back off the floor. Inhale as you slowly release down. Repeat eight times.
HELPFUL HINTS	Keep your chin off your chest and keep your neck as relaxed as possible.

Benefits abdominals

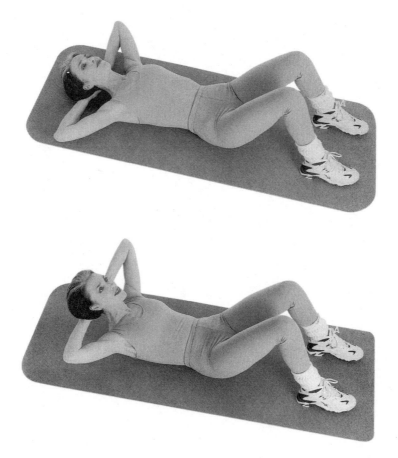

STARTING POSITION Lie on your back with your knees bent, feet flat on the floor. Clasp both hands behind your head and bring your elbows out to the side.

ACTION Exhale as you tilt your pelvis, then lift your upper back off the floor. Inhale as you slowly release down.

LEVEL 2 Do two sets of eight.

LEVEL 3 Do two sets of ten.

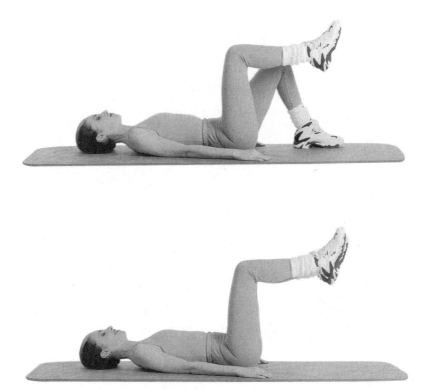

STARTING POSITION	Lie on your back with both knees bent, feet flat on the floor, arms along sides. Press lower back into the ground (pelvic tilt) and bring your right knee in to your chest.
ACTION	Inhale as you lift your left knee in to your chest to meet your right. Exhale as you lower your right foot down, then left foot down. Repeat eight times.
HELPFUL HINT	Keep your abdomen flat and your pelvis still to keep your lower back from arching.
LEVEL 2	Do two sets of eight.
LEVEL 3	Do two sets of ten.

Benefits abdominals and obliques (waist)

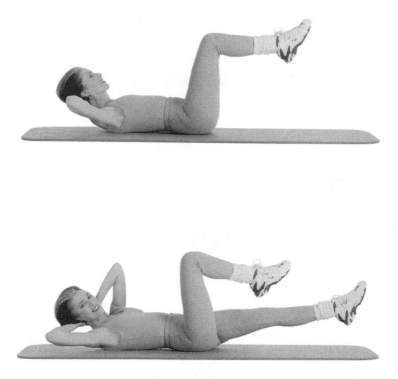

STARTING POSITION	Lie on your back with both knees bent and hands behind your head. Bring both knees in to your chest as you lift your head and upper back off the floor.
ACTION	Twist torso toward the right knee as you extend the left leg out. Then twist torso toward the left knee as you extend the right leg out. Repeat eight times on each side.
HELPFUL HINT	Take a breath during each extension.
LEVEL 2	Do two sets of eight.
LEVEL 3	Do two sets of ten.

Benefits erector spinae (muscles on both sides of spine)

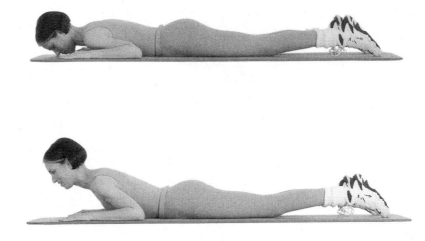

STARTING POSITION	Lie on your stomach with your hands by your head, elbows bent at right angles and forearms on the floor, head down.
ACTION	Exhale as you press your hand into the floor and raise your chest, until you're arching slightly. Hold for three counts, then inhale as you release down. Repeat eight times.
HELPFUL HINTS	Keep your pelvis on the floor and look down while pushing up.
LEVEL 2	Do eight press-ups.
LEVEL 3	Do ten press-ups.

Benefits erector spinae and latissimus dorsi (back)

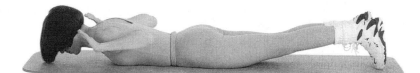

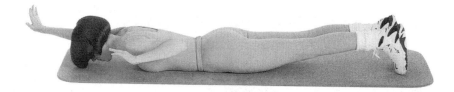

STARTING POSITION	Lie on your stomach with your hands by your head, elbows bent at right angles and forearms on the floor, head down. Push onto the balls of your feet so both knees are off the floor. Press your shoulder blades together and lift your arms off the floor.
ACTION	Alternate, pushing your right arm and then your left arm straight out in front of your head. Repeat five times, alternating arms.
HELPFUL HINT	Breathe naturally throughout the exercise.
LEVEL 2	Do eight pushes with each arm, alternating.
LEVEL 3	Do ten pushes with each arm, alternating.

Benefits erector spinae and lower back

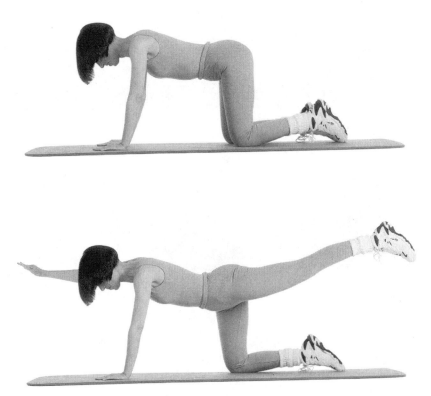

STARTING POSITION	Start on your hands and knees, facedown.
ACTION	Exhale as you extend and lift your right arm and left leg. Head remains facing down as you hold for three seconds; inhale and lower. Repeat eight times, alternating sides.
LEVEL 2	Repeat eight times, alternating sides.
LEVEL 3	Repeat ten times, alternating sides.

FLEXIBILITY COOLDOWN

Hold each stretch for ten to thirty seconds

QUADRICEP STRETCH Lie on your stomach, face down. Bend your right knee behind you and grab hold of your foot. Bring your heel toward your buttocks, as close as possible without straining, while breathing deeply. Slowly release down. Repeat with left leg.

BACK STRETCH Lie on your stomach facedown. Use your hands to press up and back onto your heels, bending your knees. Stretch your arms and fingers in front of you on the floor, stretching out your back.

HAMSTRING STRETCH Turn onto your back. Bend both knees and place your feet flat on the floor. Bend your right knee in to your chest, then extend the leg straight up, keeping both hips on the floor. If you want additional stretch, you can wrap both hands around your thigh and gently pull the leg in toward your body. Release by bending your knee, then lowering it to floor. Repeat with left leg.

CHEST STRETCH Roll onto one side, then use your hands to help yourself up to standing. Go into a doorway and hold on to the sides with your elbows bent at 90-degree angles. Step forward with one leg, as if you're walking into the room, so that your elbows are slightly behind you and your chest is open.

NECK AND SHOULDER STRETCH Stand tall, then tilt your head to the left side and the right. Extend your right arm up and stretch; then stretch your left arm. Roll your shoulders back a few times. Shake out any spots that feel tight.

LIFESTYLE LIFTS

ENJOY HEALTHY ENERGY SNACKS Now that you're exercising more often, you may be working up a bigger appetite. Instead of having sugary and fatty foods that slow you down, buy yourself an assortment of nutritious snacks:

- Fresh fruits and juices
- Raw vegetables
- Nuts, seeds, and dried fruits
- Whole grain breads and bagels
- Air-popped popcorn and pretzels

Remember, *small* portions are recommended, both for maintaining your energy level and for weight concerns. You may want to eat larger portions of raw vegetables and fruits than nuts, seeds, and breads. Be sensible about your portions and eat slowly and consciously.

Let's face it, baby carrots may never replace chocolate chip cookies in your heart. But you can learn to make the healthy choices a *habit* and the high-fat foods a special treat instead of vice versa. You can reduce your cravings for foods with high sugar and fat content and learn to appreciate natural snacks.

REDUCE YOUR INTAKE OF SUGAR, CAFFEINE, AND ALCOHOL

This step goes hand-in-hand with the preceding Lifestyle Lift. The goal is gradually to establish habits that nourish you, and reduce or eliminate ones that deplete your resources.

If you are menopausal, you have extra motivation to reduce your intake of sugar, caffeine, and alcohol since these substances can trigger hot flashes. They can also exacerbate mood swings, anxiety, fatigue, and sleeplessness in women of all ages.

This week, try a new approach: Substitute exercise and/or healthy snacks for the substances you use to cope with stress, fatigue, anxiety, boredom, and other difficult feelings. Here are ways to put this plan into action:

▸ Bring small snacks of fruit, crudités, nuts, seeds, or air-popped popcorn to work so you're not at the·mercy of the donut cart or vending machines.
▸ Take a mid-morning stretching break instead of a coffee and donut break. Have a healthy snack after you loosen up and relax.
▸ After lunch and dinner, eat fresh fruit to satisfy your craving for a sweet dessert.
▸ Drink fruit juice mixed with club soda or seltzer as a substitute for sweetened, caffeinated sodas.
▸ Try herbal teas and coffee substitutes made from grains.
▸ Instead of relying on caffeine or sugar to counteract your afternoon slump, take a walk or do some stretching for a burst of energy.
▸ Instead of having alcoholic drinks to relax after a hard day, do your favorite aerobic exercise or the Strength Training Routine.
▸ Set up exercise dates with friends instead of meeting at bars and restaurants. Or work out before going out. If you exercise first, you'll be less likely to overindulge in food and drink.
▸ If you have an addiction to alcohol, drugs, or nicotine, or an eating disorder, you should seek professional help or peer support.

PRACTICE A RELAXATION TECHNIQUE

Another way to support your efforts to overcome unhealthy habits is to practice conscious relaxation techniques.

This week, select one of the do-it-yourself relaxation exercises in Chapter 10: deep breathing, autogenic training, or progressive relaxation. Read through the exercise a few times, then lie down in a quiet place and try it. Don't expect to achieve complete concentration and relaxation the first time; just go with the flow and enjoy the soothing effect. Practice the same method again later in the week.

If you're interested in delving deeper into relaxation methods, you might also read a book or take a class to learn meditation or yoga. Biofeedback, which is taught in a clinical setting, is another option you can explore.

CONTINUE WITH YOUR EFFORTS FROM WEEK 1

As you add new Lifestyle Lifts each week of the program, continue the efforts you started earlier. This allows the program to go beyond being an exercise regime—it can be a time of total mind/body renewal and growth.

In Week 2, continue with your Week 1 Lifestyle Lifts:

- ‣ Increase your calcium intake
- ‣ Drink six to eight glasses of water daily
- ‣ Pay attention to improving your posture

CHECKLIST FOR WEEK 2

1. Write down appointments for aerobic exercise and the Strength Training Routine.
2. Do an Aerobic Activity at least three times during the week for the duration listed in the chart for your fitness level. Include warm-up and cooldown.
3. Do the Strength Training Routine twice this week.
4. Substitute natural energy foods for snacks with high sugar and fat content.
5. Take steps to reduce your intake of sugar, caffeine, and alcohol.
6. Try a conscious relaxation technique twice this week.
7. Continue with the Lifestyle Lifts from Week 1.

WEEK 3 OF THE 4-WEEK WORKOUT PROGRAM

Start this week of the program by writing down your exercise appointments: three days of Aerobic Activity and two days of the Strength Training Routine for strength and flexibility.

Continue with your favorite form of aerobics for two of the sessions and try a different activity at least once. This allows you to see progress in your main fitness form while you also expand your exercise repertoire.

One morning this week, take a few minutes to determine your Target Heart Rate (THR) zone, using the Karvonen Formula in Chapter 6. Later that day, during a session of your regular Aerobic Activity, pause after about ten minutes. Measure your heart rate by counting your pulse and checking your watch for ten seconds. Your heart rate should fall somewhere in your THR zone. If it's higher, reduce the intensity of your aerobic workout; if it's lower, you may need to step up the pace to gain cardiorespiratory advantages.

In between aerobic days, you'll be doing the third Strength Training Routine. By now you may be familiar enough with the warm-up and cooldown movements to perform them without reading the instructions. The photographs will guide you through the new muscle-strength exercises.

WARM-UP

▸ ▸

FOR HEAD AND SHOULDERS
▸ ▸ ▸ ▸ ▸ ▸ ▸ ▸ ▸ ▸ ▸

STARTING POSITION   Stand with your legs slightly apart, knees soft. Check your posture: shoulders should be relaxed, spine long, weight to your heels. Breathe deeply into your abdomen.

ACTION   Inhale and bring your arms up to the sides and overhead. Exhale and soften your knees as you bring your arms down. Repeat eight times, up and down.

Tilt your head to the right side, down to center, and left. Reverse, making three slow-half circles to each side.

Roll your right shoulder back, then your left shoulder back, four times. Add a lunge, right side and left side, as you're rolling your shoulders. Repeat eight times.

FOR UPPER BACK
▸ ▸ ▸ ▸ ▸ ▸ ▸ ▸ ▸ ▸

STARTING POSITION   Stand tall with your legs hip-width apart.

ACTION   Lift your arms to the sides. Bend your knees and bring your arms and upper back forward as if you're hugging a big beach ball. Inhale and open your arms out to the sides as you straighten your legs. Repeat four times.

Place your hands on top of your thighs and bend your knees, turn your toes out slightly and bend your torso forward. Reach your right shoulder forward and look up to the left. Hold ten seconds and breathe. Switch to the other side and hold ten seconds. Repeat four times on each side.

Keep your knees bent and toes forward. Inhale and curl your tailbone under. Exhale and extend your tailbone toward the ceiling. Repeat three times. Keep your knees bent, slowly roll up.

FOR FULL BODY
▸ ▸ ▸ ▸ ▸ ▸ ▸ ▸ ▸ ▸

STARTING POSITION   Stand tall.

ACTION   Walk in place. Punch your arms forward, to the sides, and overhead, eight times in each direction. Do two times through.

STRENGTH EXERCISES
▸ ▸

NOTE: The starting position and action for all three levels are the same on the following muscle-strength-building exercises. The repetitions in the initial *Action* section are for Level 1. However, additional sets, repetitions, and/or weights are given for Levels 2 and 3. Women with low bone density/osteoporosis, please refer to the strength workout in Chapter 17.

Benefits pectorals (chest), triceps (back of arms)

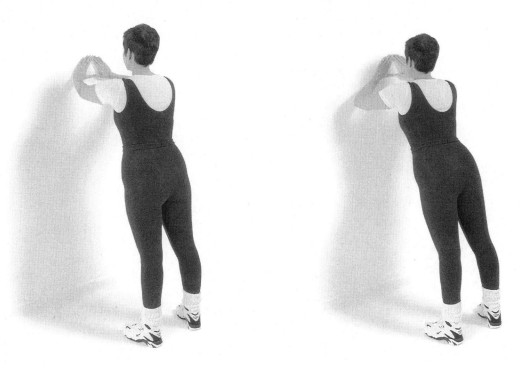

STARTING POSITION Standing, place both hands on the wall; the thumbs and forefingers of each hand should meet, forming a triangle hold.

ACTION Inhale and bend your elbows as you lean in to the wall. Exhale and push out until your arms are straight. Repeat eight times.

LEVEL 2 Do two sets of eight wall pushups.

(LEVEL 3) MODIFIED PUSHUP

Benefits pectorals (chest), triceps (back of arms)

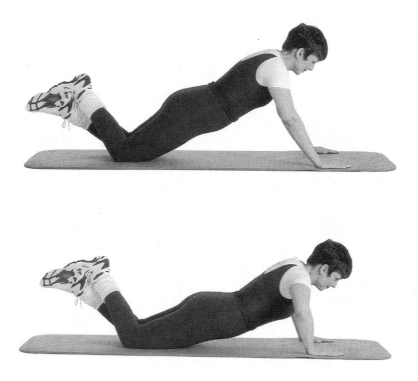

STARTING POSITION Start on your hands and knees facedown, with ankles crossed and arms straight.

ACTION Inhale and bend your elbows as you lower yourself almost to the floor. Exhale and push out until your arms are straight. Do two sets of ten.

Benefits rhomboids (mid-back), latissimus dorsi (back), biceps (front of arms)

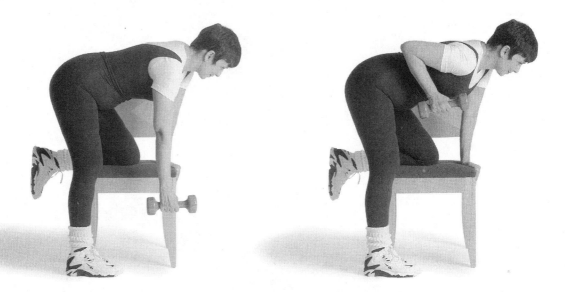

STARTING POSITION Stand beside a couch or chair. Rest your left knee and hand on it. Back is parallel to the floor, head down. Hold your 3-lb. weight in your right hand, extending right arm down.

ACTION Exhale as you bend your right elbow, bringing your arm up so your elbow is above your back. Inhale as you bring your arm down. Pull up and release down eight times with right arm, then switch sides and do eight times with the left arm.

HELPFUL HINT Use your back muscles for the lift (your shoulder blade should move with the action).

LEVEL 2 Do two sets of eight on each side, using 5-lb. weights.

LEVEL 3 Do two sets of ten on each side, using 8-lb. weights.

▸ ▸

Benefits gluteus maximus (buttocks) and abductors (outer thigh)

NOTE:
The following three exercises can be done consecutively while lying on the left side, then repeated on your right; or you can switch sides for each exercise.

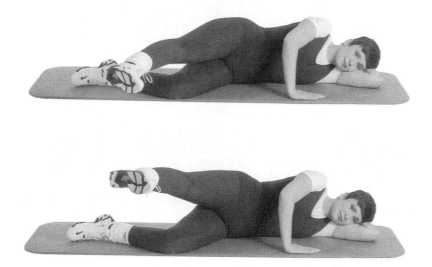

STARTING POSITION	Lie on your left side with your left knee bent and right leg extended, head relaxed on your arm. Rest your right hand about six inches in front of your body for balance. Bring your right leg forward, at a 45-degree angle from the hip joint.
ACTION	Exhale as you lift your leg. Inhale as you lower your leg down. Do two sets of eight, then repeat on the other side.
HELPFUL HINTS	Keep both hips facing forward and top leg parallel to the floor. Leg should not go higher than a 45-degree angle from the floor.
LEVEL 2	Use 3-lb. ankle weights on ankles or above your knee. Do two sets of eight.
LEVEL 3	Use 5-lb. ankle weights on ankles or above your knee. Do two sets of ten.

Benefits adductors (inner thighs)

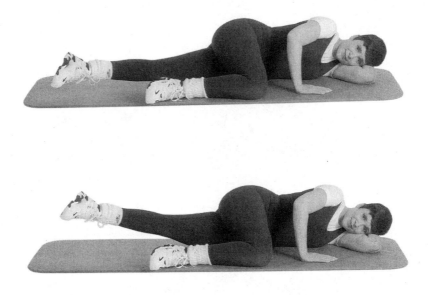

STARTING POSITION   Lie on your left side with your left leg straight, right knee bent and resting on the floor in front of you, head relaxed on your arm. Rest your right hand about six inches from your chest for balance. Lift your left leg off the floor.

ACTION   Keep your left leg lifted and pulse eight times; then lower your leg. Do another set of eight pulses, then repeat on the other side.

LEVEL 2   Use 3-lb. weights on ankles or above the knee. Do two sets of eight.

LEVEL 3   Use 5-lb. weights on ankles or above the knee. Do two sets of ten.

WING-OUT

Benefits rotator cuff (shoulder joint) and posterior deltoid (back of shoulders)

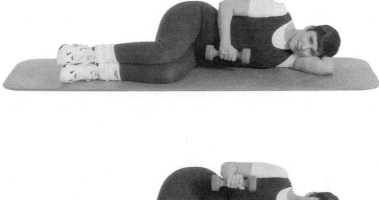

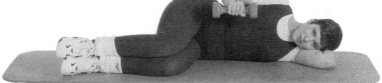

STARTING POSITION	Lie on your left side with both knees bent, right elbow resting on your hip. Hold your 3-lb. weight in your right hand, in front of your navel, palm down.
ACTION	Keeping your elbow touching your side, exhale and lift the weight toward ceiling; then inhale and lower down to navel. Repeat ten times on each side.
LEVEL 2	Do two sets of eight, using 3-lb. weights.
LEVEL 3	Do two sets of ten, using 5-lb. weights.

Benefits abdominal and sphincter muscles

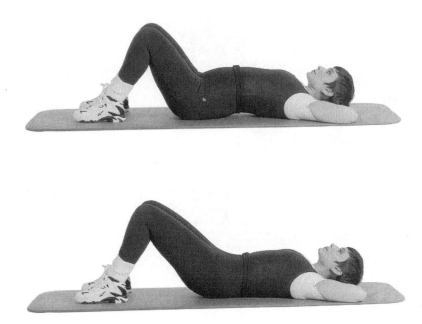

STARTING POSITION	Lie on your back with your knees bent and feet flat on the floor.
ACTION	Inhale, filling up your abdomen. Exhale and gently push your lower back into the floor while tightening your sphincter muscles. Hold for three seconds, then release. Repeat ten times.
HELPFUL HINT	As you exhale, your lower back will flatten into the floor.
LEVEL 2	Same.
LEVEL 3	Same.

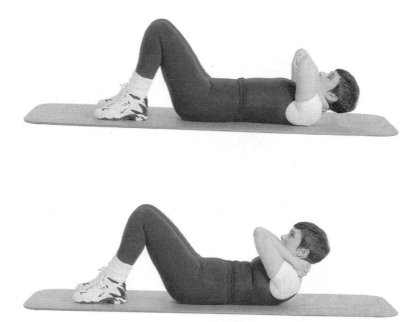

7 CURL-UPS WITH PULSES

Benefits abdominals

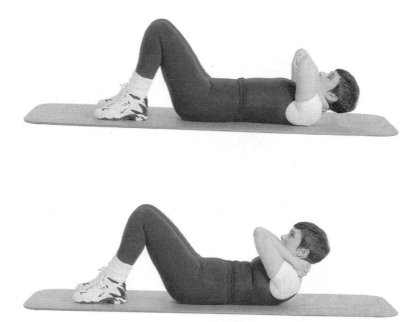

STARTING POSITION   Lie on your back with your knees bent, feet flat on the floor. Clasp both hands behind your neck and bring your elbows forward. Tilt your pelvis, then lift your upper back only off the floor.

ACTION   Stay lifted and pulse eight times, exhaling on each upward movement. Slowly lower and relax, then tilt and repeat for eight more pulses.

HELPFUL HINTS   Keep your chin off your chest and keep your neck as relaxed as possible.

Levels 2 and 3 continued on page 138

7 (LEVELS 2 AND 3) CURL-UPS WITH PULSES

▶ ▶

Benefits abdominals

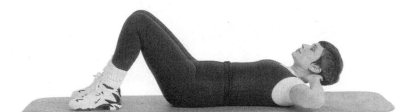

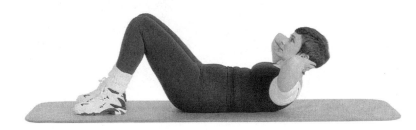

STARTING POSITION   Lie on your back with your knees bent, feet flat on the floor. Clasp both hands behind your head and bring your elbows out to the sides. Tilt your pelvis, then lift your upper back only off the floor.

ACTION   Stay lifted and pulse eight times, exhaling on each upward movement. Slowly lower and relax.

LEVEL 2   Do one more set of eight pulses (a total of two sets).

LEVEL 3   Do two sets of ten.

Benefits abdominals

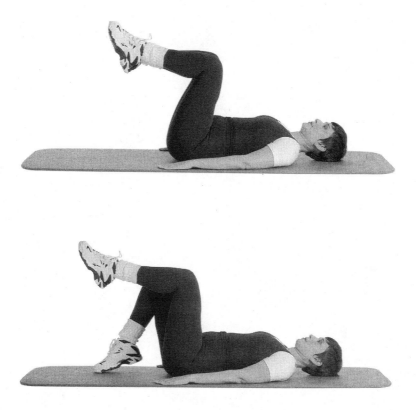

STARTING POSITION	Lie on your back with both knees bent, feet flat on the floor, arms along sides. Lift both knees in to your chest.
ACTION	Keeping both knees bent, tap your right toe on the floor, then left, alternating. Take a breath on each movement. Do eight times on each side, alternating.
HELPFUL HINT	Maintain a pelvic tilt throughout the exercise.
LEVEL 2	Do two sets of eight.
LEVEL 3	Do two sets of ten.

Benefits abdominals and obliques (waist)

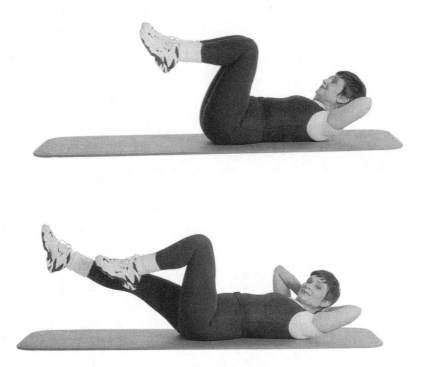

STARTING POSITION   Lie on your back with both knees bent, hands behind your head. Bring both knees in to your chest as you lift your head and upper back off the floor.

ACTION   Twist torso toward the left knee as you extend right leg out. Then twist torso toward the right knee as you extend left leg out. Repeat eight times on each side.

HELPFUL HINT   Take a breath during each extension.

LEVEL 2   Do two sets of eight.

LEVEL 3   Do two sets of ten.

Benefits erector spinae (muscles on sides of spine)

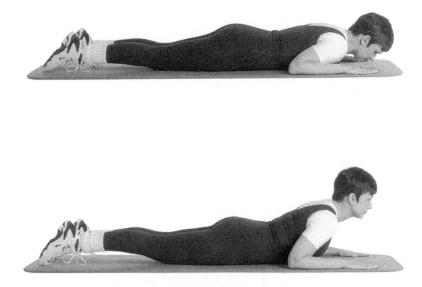

STARTING POSITION	Lie on your stomach with your hands by your head, elbows bent at right angles and forearms on the floor, head down.
ACTION	Exhale as you press your hands into the floor and raise your chest until you're arching slightly. Hold for three counts, then inhale as you release down. Repeat eight times.
HELPFUL HINTS	Keep your pelvis on the floor and look down while pushing up.
LEVEL 2	Do eight press-ups.
LEVEL 3	Do ten press-ups.

Benefits erector spinae

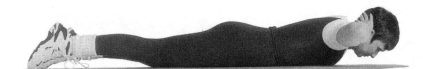

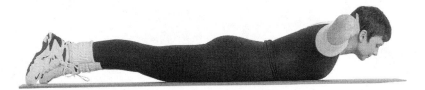

STARTING POSITION	Lie on your stomach with your hands behind your head, fingertips lightly touching.
ACTION	Exhale as you lift your upper body, pressing your shoulder blades together. Hold for three counts, then inhale as you release down. Do eight times.
HELPFUL HINT	Keep looking down to prevent arching your neck.
LEVEL 2	Do two sets of eight.
LEVEL 3	Do two sets of ten.

Benefits erector spinae and lower back

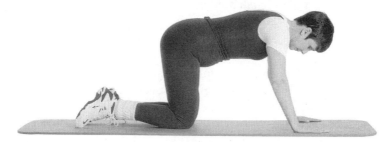

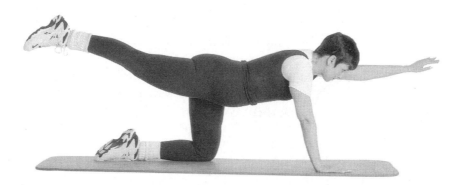

STARTING POSITION	Start on your hands and knees, facedown.
ACTION	Exhale as you extend and lift your left arm and right leg. Head remains facing down as you hold for three seconds, then inhale lower. Repeat eight times, alternating sides.
LEVEL 2	Repeat eight times, alternating sides.
LEVEL 3	Repeat ten times, alternating sides.

FLEXIBILITY COOLDOWN

Hold each stretch for ten to thirty seconds.

QUADRICEP STRETCH — Lie on your stomach, facedown. Bend your right knee behind you and grab hold of your foot. Bring your heel toward your buttocks, as close as possible without straining, while breathing deeply. Slowly release down. Repeat with left leg.

BACK STRETCH — Lie on your stomach, face down. Use your hands to press up and back onto your heels, bending your knees. Stretch your arms and fingers in front of you on the floor, stretching out your back.

HAMSTRING STRETCH — Turn onto your back. Bend both knees and place your feet flat on the floor. Bend your right knee in to your chest, then extend the leg straight up, keeping both hips on the floor. If you want additional stretch, you can wrap both hands around your thigh and gently pull the leg in toward your body. Release by bending your knee, then lowering it to floor. Repeat with left leg.

CHEST STRETCH — Roll onto one side, then use your hands to help yourself up to standing. Go into a doorway and hold on to the sides with your elbows bent at 90-degree angles. Step forward with one leg, as if you're walking into the room, so that your elbows are slightly behind you and your chest is open.

NECK AND SHOULDER STRETCH — Stand tall, then tilt your head to the left side and the right. Extend your right arm up and stretch; then stretch your left arm. Roll your shoulders back a few times. Shake out any spots that feel tight.

LIFESTYLE LIFTS

TRY DIFFERENT ENERGY ENTREES — Now that you're familiar with energy snacks, you might be encouraged to experiment with entrees. This week, try two or three new low-fat dishes for lunch and dinner.

If you like to cook, you can find a versatile selection of health-conscious cookbooks at your local bookstore or library. Take home a couple of books that have appealing recipes to try.

If you don't have a great deal of interest in cooking or the time for it, you can find prepared entrees at health food stores and better supermarkets. These include quick-cooking grains and low-fat frozen entrees. You can also have simple meals of steamed vegetables, salads, and broiled fish.

If you eat out, there are a number of ways you can stay with your low-fat, high-energy eating plan:

- Select raw fruits and vegetables at the salad bar, not foods with heavy sauces.
- Ask the server to put salad dressings, sauces, and gravies on the side, and use just a touch.
- If you're dining out, order a broiled or grilled fish or poultry entree — limit the meat. Cut down on butter and sauces on side dishes.
- You can request dishes at Chinese restaurants without thick sauces or deep frying. Many other types of ethnic restaurants also offer low-fat options; select consciously.

As part of your ongoing effort to give yourself good nutritional support, continue with the changes you began in Weeks 1 and 2:

- Have energy snacks instead of sugary, fatty foods.
- Cut down on your caffeine, alcohol, and sugar consumption.
- Drink lots of water to cleanse your system.
- Eat calcium-rich foods each day and take appropriate supplements.

GET YOURSELF SOME NEW GEAR With all these virtuous efforts, you certainly deserve a reward. How about some shopping? Treat yourself to a piece of exercise gear or clothing that will add a little splash to your workout sessions. You don't need to spend a lot of money, just be bold. Some ideas:

A warm-up suit
A leotard in a flattering style
A pair of patterned leggings or tights
A workout video
New music for exercising

If you have the means to splurge, you might shop around for a health club membership. Or you can look into purchasing equipment for a home gym. Exercise bikes, treadmills, steppers, sliders, rowing or skiing machines — the options run the gamut. Just be certain you're committed to using the machine, to avoid being saddled with a neglected piece of equipment that makes you feel guilty. If you're not certain, a trial membership at a well-equipped gym may be a better idea.

HAVE AN EXERCISE DATE One of the best ways to avoid becoming bored with exercise is to do it with someone special. In these days when everyone is so busy, exercise dates are a great way to accomplish two things at once: a social visit and a workout.

This week, plan at least one exercise date with a friend or relative. You can take a fast and friendly walk with a neighbor, a romantic bike ride with the one you love, or a challenging aerobics class with a friend.

Exercise dates are also a terrific way to break into a new sport or activity you want to try. A more experienced friend can show you the ropes, or, if you're both beginners, you can learn together and have a laugh. A partner can help you keep the right perspective: Exercise is essentially play for grown-ups, not competition.

CHECKLIST FOR WEEK 3

1. Write down your exercise appointments.
2. Do three sessions of aerobic exercise (two different activities). Measure your heart rate to see if you're working out in your Target Heart Rate zone. Warm up and cool down each time.
3. Do the third Strength Training Routine twice this week.
4. Try several low-fat, nourishing entrees. Continue with the nutritional steps of the previous weeks.
5. Reward yourself with a new piece of exercise clothing or equipment.
6. Plan an exercise date with someone whose company you enjoy.
7. Congratulate yourself on three weeks of working out consistently. Take a minute to think about the benefits.

WEEK 4 OF THE 4-WEEK WORKOUT PROGRAM

By this fourth week, it should already be a part of your routine to write down your exercise appointments: at least three sessions of aerobic exercise and two days of the Strength Training Routine. While you're doing aerobics this week, check your pulse about ten minutes into the activity to see if you're in your THR zone. After you do this a few times, you'll become more sensitive to your heart rate and be able to work at optimal intensity.

If you're feeling comfortable with your Aerobic Activity, you can also add a few minutes of higher intensity movement. For example, if you're walking, move into a slow jog for a few minutes in the middle of the session or walk up a hill. If you're biking, add an uphill sprint. Then resume your normal intensity. Never stop abruptly after working in a higher intensity; always cool down with a slower pace.

By now you may be familiar enough with the Warmup and Flexibility Cooldown sequences to concentrate on your form and breathing as you stretch. As you perform the strength exercises, you can focus on the quality of your movement and your progress.

FOR HEAD AND SHOULDERS

STARTING POSITION Stand with your legs slightly apart, knees soft. Check your posture: shoulders should be relaxed, spine long, weight to your heels. Breathe deeply into your abdomen.

ACTION Inhale and bring your arms up to the sides and overhead. Exhale and soften your knees as you bring your arms down. Repeat eight times, up and down.

Tilt your head to the right side, down to center, and left. Reverse, making three slow half-circles to each side.

Roll your right shoulder back, then your left shoulder back, four times. Add a lunge, right side and left side, as you're rolling your shoulders. Repeat eight times.

FOR UPPER BACK

STARTING POSITION Stand tall with your legs hip-width apart.

ACTION Lift your arms to the sides. Bend your knees and bring your arms and upper back forward as if you're hugging a big beach ball. Inhale and open your arms out to the sides as you straighten your legs. Repeat four times.

Place your hands on top of your thighs and bend your knees, turn your toes out slightly and bend your torso forward. Reach your right shoulder forward and look up to the left. Hold ten seconds and breathe. Switch to the other side and hold ten seconds. Repeat four times on each side.

Keep your knees bent and toes forward. Inhale and curl your tailbone under. Exhale and extend your tailbone toward the ceiling. Repeat three times. Keep your knees bent and slowly roll up.

FOR FULL BODY

STARTING POSITION Stand tall.

ACTION Walk in place. Punch your arms forward, to the sides, and overhead, eight times in each direction. Do two times through.

STRENGTH EXERCISES

▸ ▸

NOTE: The starting position and action for all three levels are the same on the following muscle-strength-building exercises. The repetitions in the initial *Action* section are for Level 1. However, additional sets, repetitions and/or weights are given for Levels 2 and 3. Women with low bone density/osteoporosis, please refer to the muscle strength/endurance workout in Chapter 17.

1 | WALL SLIDE

▸ ▸

Benefits quadriceps (front of thighs) and hamstrings (back of thighs), abdominals

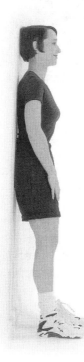 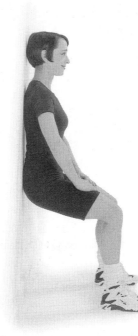

STARTING POSITION	Stand with your back against a wall and your feet parallel, about twelve inches from the wall. Place your hands on your thighs.
ACTION	Slide your back down the wall (as if you're going to sit down) until your knees almost reach a 90-degree angle. Hold for three counts; then slowly slide up. Repeat eight times. Breathe naturally throughout the movement.
HELPFUL HINTS	Your knees should remain over your heels to prevent knee pain. Try to keep your lower back against the wall.
LEVEL 2	Two sets of eight.
LEVEL 3	Two sets of ten.

▶ ▶ ▶ ▶ ▶ ▶ ▶ ▶ ▶ ▶ ▶ ▶ ▶ ▶ ▶ ▶ ▶ ▶ ▶ ▶

Benefits biceps (front of arms)

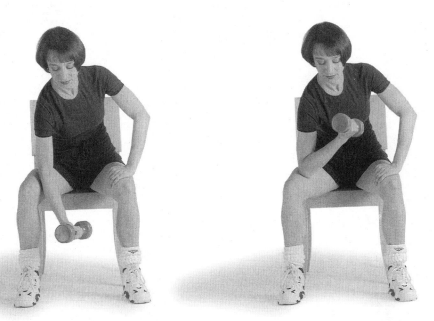

STARTING POSITION Sit on the edge of a chair or couch with legs apart. Hold a 3-lb. weight in your right hand, palm up, with your right elbow on the inside of your right thigh. Support your body with your left hand resting on your left thigh.

ACTION Exhale as you bend your elbow, bringing the weight up toward your shoulder. Inhale and slowly release down. Repeat eight times, then repeat on the other side.

HELPFUL HINT Keep your working arm pressing against your inner thigh.

LEVEL 2 Do two sets of eight, using 5-lb. weights.

LEVEL 3 Do two sets of ten, using 8-lb. weights.

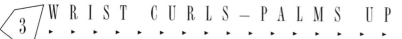
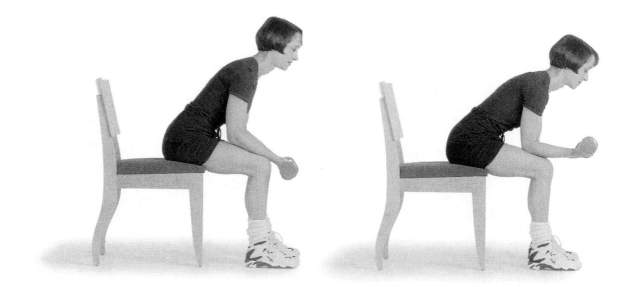

STARTING POSITION   Sit on the edge of a couch or chair, feet flat on the floor. Rest your forearms on top of your thighs, palms up, holding 3-lb. weights.

ACTION   Exhale and curl your wrists in; inhale, extend out. Repeat eight times.

LEVEL 2   Do two sets of eight, using 5-lb. weights.

LEVEL 3   Do two sets of ten, using 5-lb. weights.

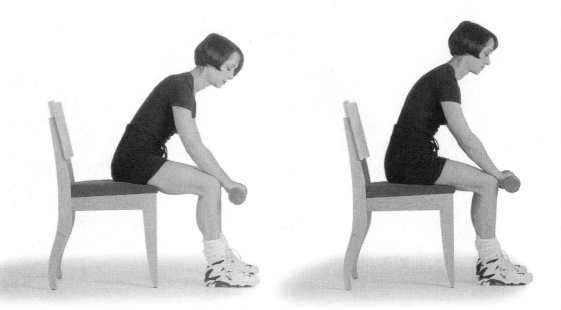

STARTING POSITION Sit on the edge of a couch or chair, feet flat on the floor. Rest your forearms on top of your thighs, palms down, holding 3-lb. weights.

ACTION Exhale and curl your wrists up; inhale, lower down. Repeat eight times.

LEVEL 2 Do two sets of eight, using 5-lb. weights.

LEVEL 3 Do two sets of ten, using 5-lb. weights.

5 DIPS

Benefits triceps (back of arms)

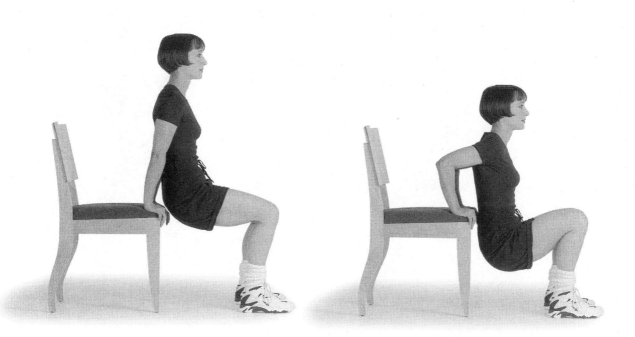

STARTING POSITION	Sit on the edge of a chair or couch, place your hands on the edge also, and your legs hip-width apart. Move your body forward so your buttocks are off the chair, weight resting on your hands and feet, knees at a 90-degree angle.
ACTION	Inhale and bend your knees and elbows as you slowly lower your buttocks nearly to the floor. Exhale as you straighten your arms and lift your buttocks. Repeat eight times.
HELPFUL HINTS	Keep your knees over your heels as you lower and lift. Keep your buttocks close to the chair.
LEVEL 2	Do two sets of eight.
LEVEL 3	Do two sets of ten, with legs extended straight out.

Benefits deltoids (shoulders)

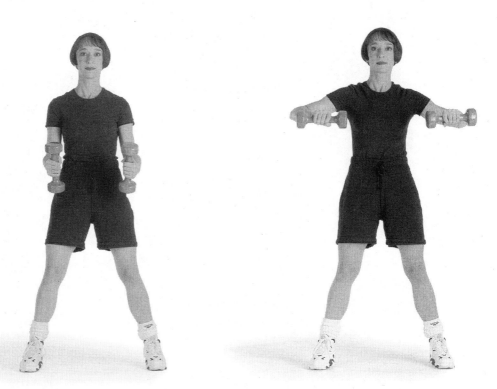

STARTING POSITION	Stand with your legs hip-width apart and knees slightly bent. Hold 3-lb. weights at your sides with your elbows bent at 90-degree angles and palms facing each other.
ACTION	Keeping your arms bent, exhale as you lift your arms toward the ceiling until they are parallel to the floor with palms facing down. Inhale and lower your arms, bringing your elbows to your sides. Do eight times.
HELPFUL HINTS	Keep your back supported by tightening your abdominal muscles and pressing your shoulders down and back.
LEVEL 2	Do two sets of eight using 5-lb. weights.
LEVEL 3	Do two sets of ten using 8-lb. weights.

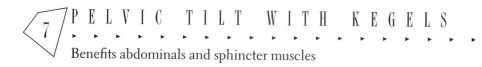
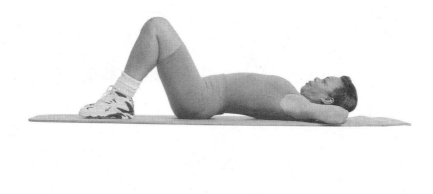

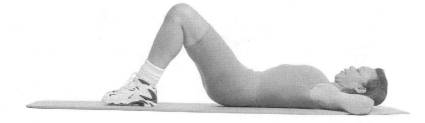

STARTING POSITION	Lie on your back with your knees bent and feet flat on the floor.
ACTION	Inhale, filling up your abdomen. Exhale and gently push your lower back into the floor while tightening your sphincter muscles. Hold for three seconds, then release. Repeat ten times.
HELPFUL HINT	As you exhale, your abdominals will flatten into the floor.
LEVEL 2	Same.
LEVEL 3	Same.

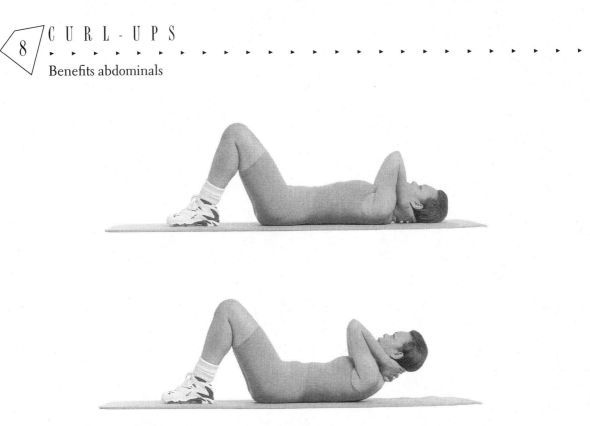

STARTING POSITION Lie on your back with your knees bent, feet flat on the floor. Clasp both hands behind your neck and bring your elbows forward.

ACTION Exhale as you tilt your pelvis and lift your upper back off the floor. Inhale as you slowly release down. Repeat eight times.

HELPFUL HINTS Keep your chin off your chest and keep your neck as relaxed as possible.

8 (LEVELS 2 AND 3) CURL-UPS

Benefits abdominals

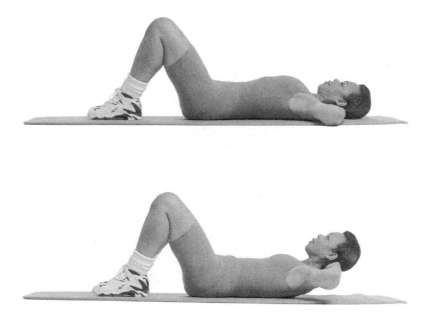

STARTING POSITION Lie on your back with your knees bent, feet flat on the floor. Clasp both hands behind your head and bring your elbows out to the side.

ACTION Exhale as you tilt your pelvis and lift your upper back off the floor. Inhale as you slowly release down.

LEVEL 2 Do two sets of eight.

LEVEL 3 Do two sets of ten.

Benefits abdominals

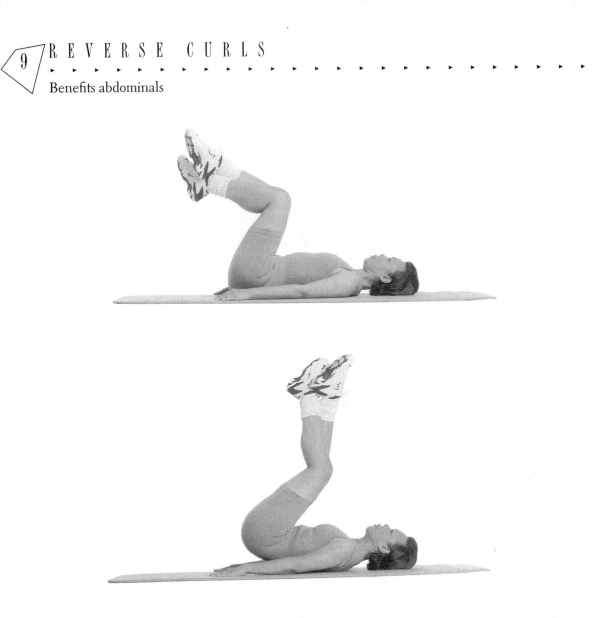

STARTING POSITION	Lie on your back with your knees bent and arms by your sides. Lift your feet off the floor, bringing your knees in to your chest, and crossing your ankles.
ACTION	Exhale and lift your lower back off the ground, curling in. Inhale as you release. Repeat eight times.
HELPFUL HINT	Do the exercise slowly, as a small movement.
LEVEL 2	Do two sets of eight.
LEVEL 3	Do two sets of ten.

Benefits abdominals and obliques (waist)

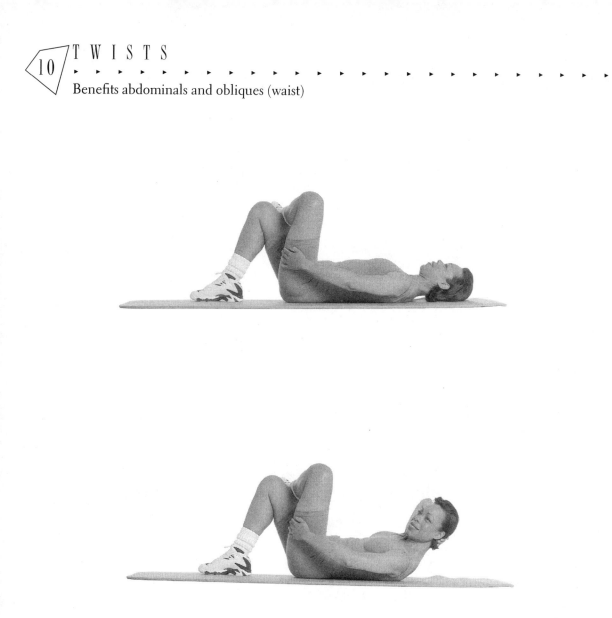

STARTING POSITION	Lie on your back with both knees bent. Cross your left foot over your right knee, letting the left knee turn out. Place your right hand behind your head and left arm holding on to the outside of your left thigh.
ACTION	Exhale as you lift yourself toward your left knee. Inhale as you slowly lower. Repeat eight times on each side.
LEVEL 2	Do two sets of eight on each side.
LEVEL 3	Do two sets of ten on each side.

PRESS-UPS II

Benefits erector spinae

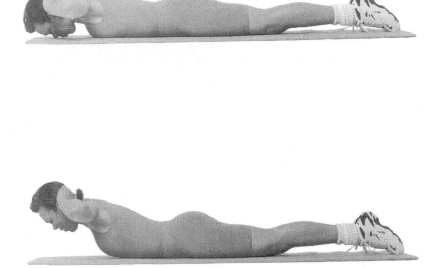

STARTING POSITION   Lie on your stomach with your hands behind your head, fingertips lightly touching.

ACTION   Exhale as you lift your upper body, pressing your shoulder blades together. Hold for three counts, then inhale as you release down. Do eight times.

HELPFUL HINT   Keep looking down to prevent arching your neck.

LEVEL 2   Do two sets of eight.

LEVEL 3   Do two sets of ten.

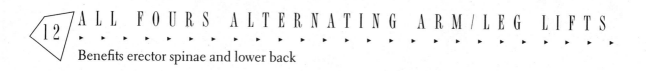
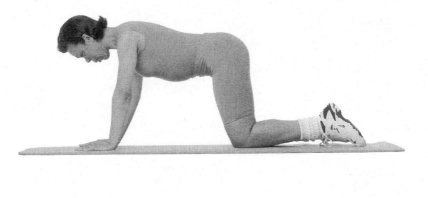

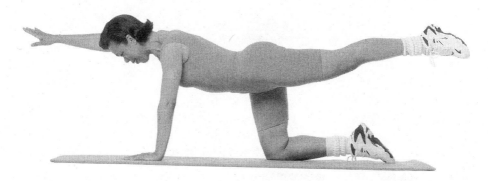

STARTING POSITION	Start on your hands and knees, facedown.
ACTION	Exhale as you extend and lift your right arm and left leg. Head remains facing down as you hold for three seconds, inhale and lower. Repeat eight times, alternating sides.
LEVEL 2	Repeat eight times, alternating sides.
LEVEL 3	Repeat ten times, alternating sides.

▶ ▶

Benefits all major muscles of the back and arms

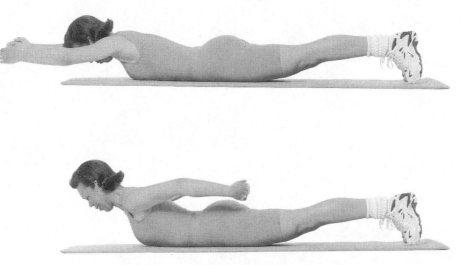

STARTING POSITION   Lie on your stomach with your arms extended overhead on the floor. Push on to the balls of your feet so both knees are off the floor. Tighten your buttocks and lift your chest and arms.

ACTION   Circle your arms behind your lower back until your hands touch. Keeping your arms straight and lifted, circle your arms forward until your hands touch in front of you. Breathe on each movement. Repeat eight times.

HELPFUL HINT   Keep facing down but keep your arms lifted throughout the movement.

LEVEL 2   Do two sets of eight.

LEVEL 3   Do two sets of ten.

FLEXIBILITY COOLDOWN

Hold each stretch for ten to thirty seconds.

QUADRICEP STRETCH Lie on your stomach, facedown. Bend your right knee behind you and grab hold of your foot. Bring your heel toward your buttocks, as close as possible without straining, breathing deeply. Slowly release down. Repeat with left leg.

BACK STRETCH Lie on your stomach, facedown. Use your hands to press up and back onto your heels, bending your knees. Stretch your arms and fingers in front of you on the floor, stretching out your back.

HAMSTRING STRETCH Turn onto your back. Bend both knees and place your feet flat on the floor. Bend your right knee in to your chest, then extend the leg straight up, keeping both hips on the floor. If you want additional stretch, you can wrap both hands around your thigh and gently pull the leg in toward your body. Release by bending your knee, then lowering it to floor. Repeat with left leg.

CHEST STRETCH Roll onto one side, then use your hands to help yourself up to standing. Go into a doorway and hold on to the sides with your elbows bent at 90-degree angles. Step forward with one leg, as if you're walking into the room, so that your elbows are slightly behind you and your chest is open.

NECK AND SHOULDER STRETCH Stand tall, then tilt your head to the left side and the right. Extend your right arm up and stretch; then stretch your left arm. Roll your shoulders back a few times. Shake out any spots that feel tight.

LIFESTYLE LIFTS

ACCELERATE YOUR ENERGY EATING PLAN WITH SIX SMALL MEALS A DAY In previous weeks you've added high-energy snacks and low-fat entrees to your diet, and tried to reduce your intake of sugar, caffeine, and alcohol. You've evaluated and increased your calcium and water consumption. Hopefully, you've noticed that you feel and look better as a result of these efforts, and you're inspired to keep going.

This week you can take another step in your energy eating plan by adjusting the pattern of your meals. Instead of having three large meals a day, try eating six small ones. Instead of making dinner the largest meal, make it the smallest. If you want to lose weight, the strategy of eating less later in the day is especially effective.

There may be some days this week when you want to sit down to a full dinner with your family or friends. You don't need to be rigid in your new eating patterns or feel deprived. Just try the energy eating plan a couple of days this week and observe how you feel.

TAKE THE PLUNGE AND TRY A NEW ACTIVITY

After three weeks of progressive exercise, you've gained confidence in your physical abilities. Use this momentum to experience a new activity. It may be a popular sport that you've always admired, or a more unusual type of exercise.

Be careful, but be adventurous. Whatever your condition, you can find a variety of active pursuits that are right for you. Here are some ideas:

LEVEL 1	LEVEL 2	LEVEL 3
Aqua aerobics	Rollerblading	Mountain trekking
Tai chi chuan	Volleyball	Scuba diving
Yoga	Ballet or jazz dance classes	Hip-hop aerobics
Ballroom dancing	Canoeing	Basketball
Croquet	Ice skating	Martial arts

These guidelines are not stringent for the three fitness levels. Use your judgment and experience to make your own choices. You can get other ideas from friends, magazines, and your own imagination. A challenging physical activity will strengthen your confidence and open up your world.

CONTINUE WITH YOUR RELAXATION PRACTICE AND POSTURE IMPROVEMENT

This week, continue to practice a simple technique to induce conscious relaxation. A pleasant time to do this is after the Flexibility Cooldown, when you're loose and ready to relax completely.

You might try an experiment: In a stressful situation, take a few minutes to detach and practice deep breathing. Notice how this helps you to cope with difficult situations and emotions.

This week you can also continue to develop awareness of your posture in everyday life. How is your posture when you are sitting at your desk, talking on the telephone, carrying a package? Evaluate the elements you need to change and use your developing muscle strength to improve your posture.

INDULGE IN A SPA TREATMENT When you're working your body hard, it's delicious to indulge in a little pampering. To celebrate the fourth week of your 4-Week Workout Program, set aside a few hours for a spa treatment. There are many ways to nourish yourself; what you choose depends on your budget and personal preferences.

On the high end, you can sign up for a day of services at a spa, beauty salon, or health club. You can enjoy various types of massages, facials, herbal skin treatments, mud baths, manicures, pedicures, and hair treatments. You can be treated like Cleopatra, or like Dorothy in the Emerald City — rubbed, scrubbed, buffed, burnished, and pampered to the hilt.

If this is too extravagant, you can opt for a favorite professional treatment, such as a massage or facial. Or you can do it yourself. Here are suggestions for low-cost, at-home spa treatments:

- Exchange massages with a friend. You can learn a great deal about massage techniques from books and videos.
- Set aside a morning to take an extra-long, scented bath. Do deep breathing and gentle stretching exercises in the tub.
- After a bath or shower, massage your body with moisturizer. Use a facial mask for deep cleansing. Give yourself a pedicure and a manicure as a final touch.
- Refer to a book with recipes for herbal skin, body, and bath treatments. Prepare your potions ahead of time, then devote yourself to a natural spa session at home. You can do yoga stretches and relaxation exercises as the final step in your transformation.

CHECKLIST FOR WEEK 4
▸ ▸

1. Write down your exercise appointments: three to four days for aerobics; two sessions of the Strength Training Routine.
2. During your aerobics, check your THR zone. Try to increase your intensity slightly for a moment, then return to the normal level.
3. Bring awareness of form and breathing into the warm-up, cooldown, and strength exercises.

4. Progress in your energy eating plan, trying six small meals a day. Continue to reduce sugar, caffeine, and alcohol. Maintain increased calcium and water intake.
5. Try a new physical activity that's fun and exciting.
6. Continue with your conscious relaxation practice and posture improvement.
7. Pamper yourself with a spa treatment.

Congratulations on completing the 4-Week Workout Program for Women Over 40. *Now you can continue to exercise your way into a healthy future.*

THE WORKOUT PROGRAM FOR WOMEN WITH OSTEOPOROSIS

"Exercise has many benefits in addition to bone health. These include increased endurance, muscle strength, flexibility, coordination, balance, and improved reaction time. These benefits can help minimize the consequences of osteoporosis; for example, fracture and postural deformities."

—THERESA CHIAIA, P.T.

Senior Physical Therapist
The Sports Medicine Center, Hospital for Special Surgery, New York City

If you have been diagnosed with osteoporosis and have perhaps suffered from a fracture due to this condition, there's no reason you can't enjoy all the fun and health benefits of exercise. The aerobic suggestions and strength-training workout in this chapter will help you achieve this goal. Physical activity is not a substitute for HRT or other medications related to osteoporosis; it is an adjunct to overall health and well-being.

The workout provides a balanced strength-building routine without any twisting, forward flexion, or jarring movements. Although this routine is safe for most women with osteoporosis, it is recommended that you show your physician the exercises before starting, to be certain they are appropriate for you.

If you have low bone density, regular exercise — along with adequate calcium, vitamin D, and appropriate medical intervention — is necessary for slowing bone loss. Exercise also gives you increased stability and balance to help prevent falls and fractures. And it provides a sense of confidence and pleasure in your body that is wonderfully liberating. A diagnosis of osteoporosis can actually open up your life instead of limiting it by motivating you to explore the world of movement.

AEROBIC ACTIVITIES

▶ ▶ ▶ ▶ ▶ ▶ ▶ ▶ ▶

"In terms of an exercise program, we start by trying to find out what a patient likes to do. It may vary from a simple program of walking to low-impact aerobics to becoming involved in a sport like tennis. A couple of my patients have taken up tap dancing. Enjoying an exercise program is key to motivation and adherence to a regular schedule."

—THERESA GALSWORTHY, R.N., O.N.C.

For women with osteoporosis, the goal is to participate in a weight-bearing Aerobic Activity for a duration of thirty minutes or more, at 50 to 75 percent of maximum heart rate, three to five days a week. However, depending on your condition, you may need to build up to this level over a period of several weeks.

If you have not exercised for many years, be gentle but firm with yourself. Make a commitment to do aerobic exercise three times a week for the first two weeks of the program and four times a week for the following two weeks.

Depending on your condition, you may need to start off with less than thirty minutes of a simple activity such as walking. You can also bank your aerobic activity; for example, walk fifteen minutes in the morning and fifteen minutes in the evening to reach your thirty minutes.

Whatever aerobic activity you choose, listen to your body and don't overtax yourself at the onset. It's better to be slow and steady than to risk injury or dropout because the exercise is too difficult. And while it may be normal to have some muscle soreness or discomfort for a day or two after you start exercising, you shouldn't experience any sharp pain or muscle spasms. If you do, consult your doctor as soon as possible.

If you're not accustomed to aerobic exercise, walking outside or on a treadmill is one of the easiest ways to start. Wear walking or running shoes with good arch and heel support. If you're walking outside, carry your keys in a pocket or fanny pack rather than in a shoulder bag so you can keep your hands free and your body balanced.

As you're walking, be aware of your form: Lift your foot with each step rather than shuffling your feet. This will reduce the risk of a fall and improve your ankle strength and stability. As much as possible, walk with your head held high and your shoulder blades slightly back.

Many women with osteoporosis can safely participate in low-impact aerobic dance or step classes. If you take these classes or follow videotapes, use a low step and avoid any twisting, forward flexion, or quick, jerking movements. Know your limitations and don't push yourself too far in class. There's nothing wrong with following part of the class and walking in place during difficult or inappropriate movements.

Depending on your physical condition, you may be able to take dance classes, or use stair and cross-country skiing machines. Some women with osteoporosis are very active and have few limitations, while others need to be more careful. Again, it's safest to consult with your physician about your capabilities.

If you enjoy non-weight-bearing aerobic activities such as swimming and bicycling, it's fine to continue these pursuits, which are great for your heart and overall well-being. But as part of the Workout Program, you should add two days a week of weight-bearing aerobic activities that work the bones.

Whatever Aerobic Activity you select, warm-up and cooldown are important. The Warm-up and Flexibility Cooldown sequences framing the Strength Training Routine can be done before and after aerobics. Dance or step classes and videos should include series of warm-up and cooldown movements as well. If you're walking, swimming, or biking, you can also perform a slower version of the activity at the beginning and end of the session.

THE STRENGTH TRAINING ROUTINE

To build and maintain bone you need to work muscle. The following workout will exercise your muscles systematically and safely.

To gain any benefits, you need to do this strength workout twice a week. Each time you do the strength exercises, perform the Warm-up and Flexibility Cooldown sequences before and after.

A few of these exercises use hand-held weights and ankle weights. However, before you use the weights, do the routine without weights to get the proper form and see if you can do the exercises without pain. You should feel the exercises in the muscles you're working, but not in your spine or elsewhere. If the routine feels easy and you sense that you need more resistance, use 1- to 3-lb. weights during the exercises that mention weights.

You may want to read through the exercises and look at the photographs a few times before getting started. If you are concerned about getting up and down from the floor, you can do the lying down exercises on a firm bed. Whether you use the floor or a bed, be careful in your transitions between lying down and standing. Always get up and down by rolling onto your side and using your hands for support, to avoid forward bending.

Perform the workout in sneakers with good ankle and arch support, and tuck in the laces to avoid tripping. You can work out on a carpet or exercise mat, near a wall and a chair. Play some of your favorite music for energy and inspiration.

STARTING POSITION Stand with your legs slightly apart, knees soft. Check your posture: shoulders should be relaxed, spine long, weight to your heels. Breathe deeply into your abdomen.

ACTION Inhale and bring your arms up to the sides and overhead. Exhale and soften your knees as you bring your arms down. Repeat ten times, up and down.

Tilt your head to the right side, down to center, and left. Reverse, making three slow half circles to each side.

Roll your right shoulder back, then your left shoulder back, four times. Turn your toes out slightly and shift your weight to the right and left (a lunge) as you're rolling your shoulders. Repeat ten times.

Stand tall, then begin to walk in place. Remember to pick up your feet and keep facing forward. Punch your arms forward, to the sides, and gently overhead, ten times in each direction. Do two times through.

1 STANDING WALL PUSHUP
▸ ▸

Benefits pectorals (chest) and triceps (back of arms)

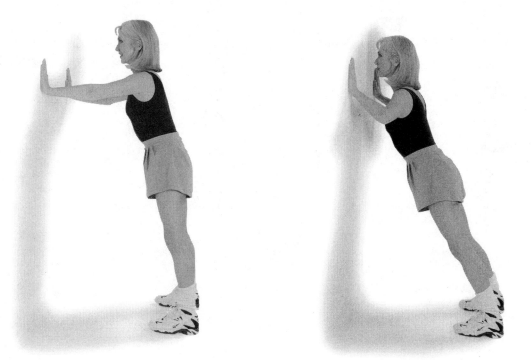

STARTING POSITION Standing, place both hands on the wall, fingertips facing up.

ACTION Inhale and bend your elbows as you lean into the wall. Exhale and push out so your arms straighten. Repeat ten wall pushups.

Benefits hamstrings (back of thighs)

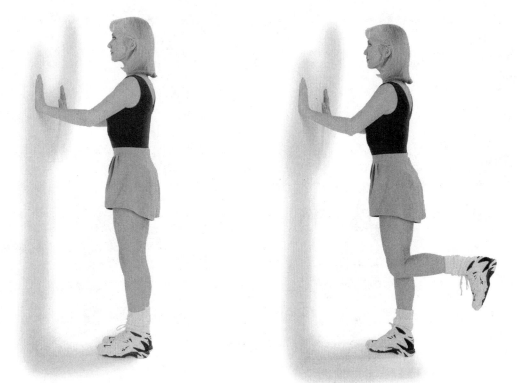

STARTING POSITION   Stand with legs hip-width apart, bend elbows slightly, and place both hands against the wall for balance.

ACTION   Exhale and bend at the knee, bringing your left heel up to your buttocks. Inhale and slowly release down. Repeat ten times on each side.

HELPFUL HINT   To make this more challenging, you can use your 1- to 3-lb. ankle weights.

Benefits rhomboids (mid-back)

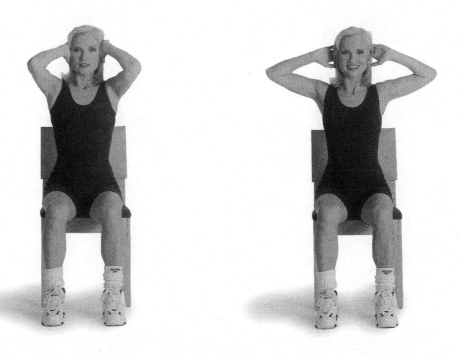

STARTING POSITION Sit on the edge of the chair, feet flat on the floor. Place your palms behind your head.

ACTION Exhale and press your shoulder blades together, bringing your elbows out to the sides. Inhale and release. Repeat ten times.

Benefits quadriceps (front of thighs)

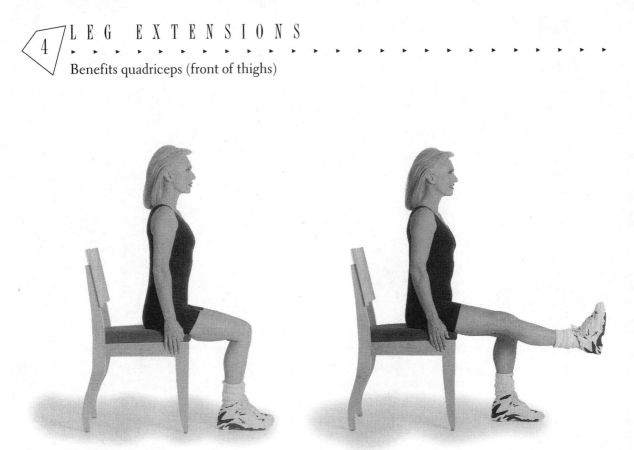

STARTING POSITION   Sit on the edge of the chair, keeping your spine long and feet flat on the floor.

ACTION   Exhale and extend your right leg; inhale and bring your leg down. Repeat ten times on each side.

HELPFUL HINTS   You can use 1- to 3-lb. ankle weights for more intensity. If more back support is needed, place a pillow behind your back.

BICEP CURLS

▸ ▸

Benefits biceps (front of arms)

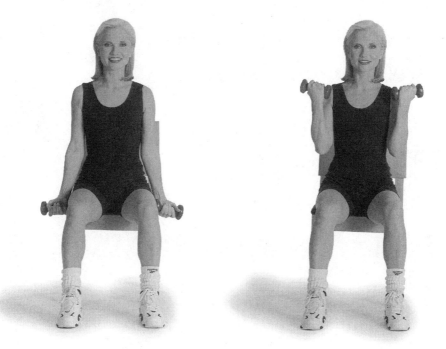

STARTING POSITION   Sit on the edge of the chair, keeping your spine long and feet flat on the floor. Hold your weights with your palms facing forward, elbows along sides.

ACTION   Exhale and bend both elbows, bringing the weights up to your shoulders. Inhale and slowly release down. Repeat ten times.

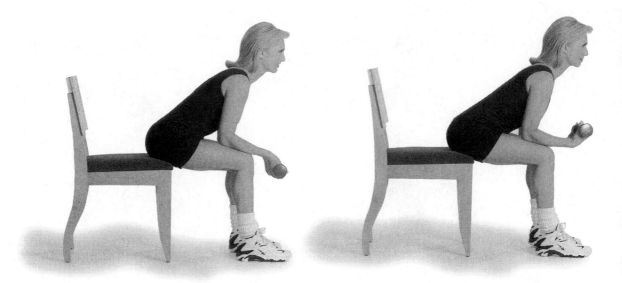

STARTING POSITION Sit on the edge of the chair, feet flat on the floor. Rest your forearms on top of your thighs with palms up, holding your weights. Your forearms will support your spine.

ACTION Exhale and curl your wrists in; inhale and extend out. Repeat ten times.

Benefits forearms and wrists

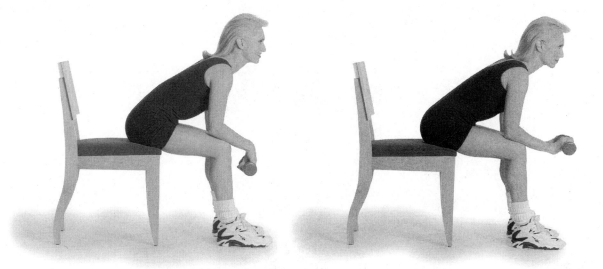

STARTING POSITION   Sit on the edge of the chair, feet flat on the floor. Rest your forearms on top of your thighs with palms down, holding your weights. Your forearms will support your spine.

ACTION   Exhale and curl your wrists up; inhale and release down. Repeat ten times.

TRANSITION TO FLOOR   You need to move to the floor from sitting without bending forward. One way to do this is to move to the edge of your chair and turn to the left. Put your right knee on the floor and slide down to your right side, using your hands for support. Then roll onto your back.

Benefits abdominals and sphincter muscles

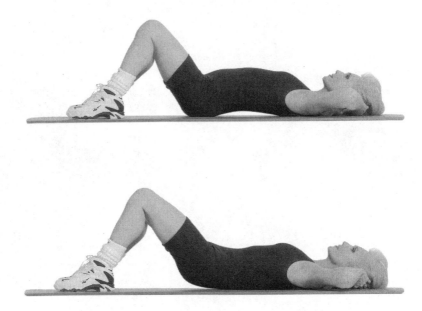

STARTING POSITION Lie on your back with your knees bent and feet flat on the floor.

ACTION Inhale, filling up your abdomen. Exhale and gently push your lower back into the floor while tightening your sphincter muscles. Hold for three seconds, then release. Repeat ten times.

HELPFUL HINT As you exhale, your abdomen will flatten into the floor.

Benefits abdominals

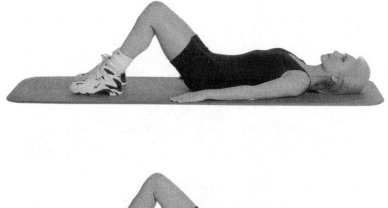

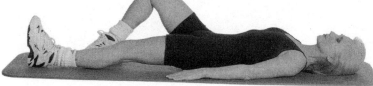

STARTING POSITION Lie on your back with your knees bent, feet flat on the floor and arms at your sides.

ACTION First, perform a pelvic tilt. Exhale while sliding one leg forward as far as you can, keeping your heel on the floor. Hold for three seconds. Maintain the pelvic tilt as you inhale and return to the starting position, then relax the tilt. Repeat with the other leg. Repeat ten times.

HELPFUL HINTS Make sure you keep your waist on the floor. To slide more easily, you can take off your sneakers and work in your socks for this and the following exercises.

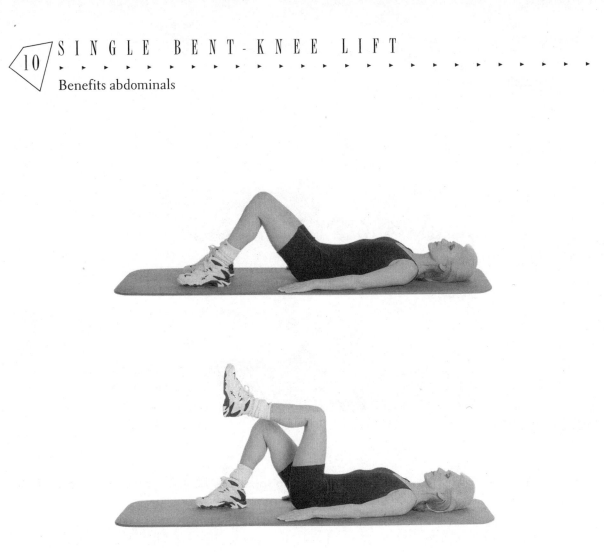
STARTING POSITION	Lie on your back with your knees bent, feet flat on the floor, and arms at your sides.
ACTION	Inhale and lift one foot off the floor, bringing your knee toward your chest. Exhale and return to starting position. Repeat on the other side. Repeat ten times.
HELPFUL HINTS	Think of pulling your abdomen up and in, as if to tuck it under your ribs. Your lower back should be flat against the floor. When you're ready to make the exercise more difficult, you can bring your thigh up to a 90-degree angle instead of all the way in to your chest.

Benefits abdominals

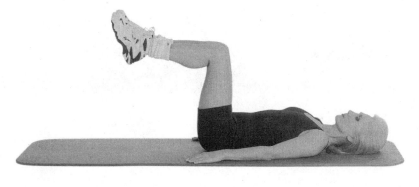

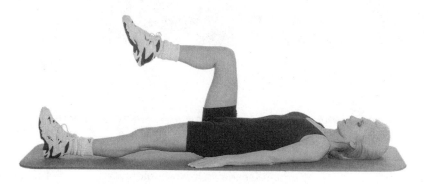

STARTING POSITION Lie on your back with your knees bent, feet flat on the floor and arms at your sides. Perform a pelvic tilt, then bring your knees in to your chest one at a time and keep them there.

ACTION Exhale and slowly slide your left leg straight down along the floor. (Your heel should make contact with the floor.) Inhale and slide your left foot back to the starting position. Repeat on the other side. Repeat ten times on each side.

HELPFUL HINT Keep your abdomen flat and your pelvis still to prevent your lower back from arching.

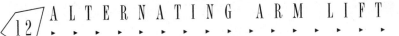

12 ALTERNATING ARM LIFT

Benefits erector spinae (muscles on both sides of spine) and lower back

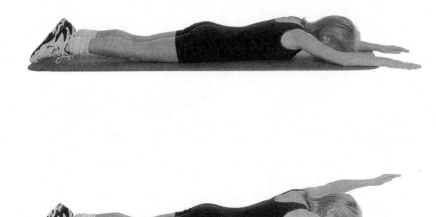

STARTING POSITION Turn onto your stomach, facedown and both arms extended on the floor.

ACTION Keeping your limbs straight, exhale as you lift your left arm. Remain facedown as you hold your arm up for three counts, inhale, and lower it. Repeat ten times, alternating sides.

Benefits gluteus (buttocks) and lower back

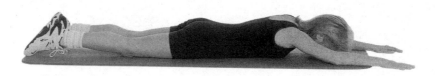

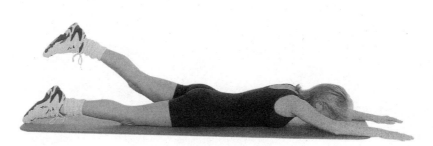

STARTING POSITION Lie on your stomach, facedown, and extend both arms overhead on the floor.

ACTION Keeping your limbs straight, exhale as you lift your left leg. Remain facedown as you hold your leg up for three counts, inhale, and lower it. Repeat ten times, alternating sides.

Benefits erector spinae and lower back

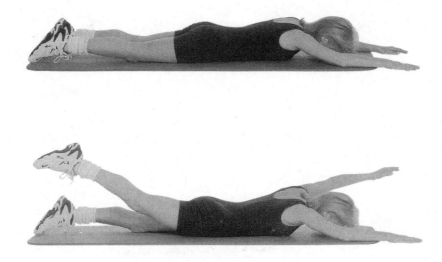

STARTING POSITION Lie on your stomach, facedown, and extend both arms overhead on the floor.

ACTION Keeping your limbs straight, exhale as you lift your left arm and right leg. Remain facedown as you hold for three counts, inhale, and lower. Repeat ten times, alternating sides.

Benefits erector spinae

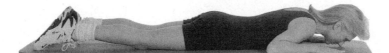

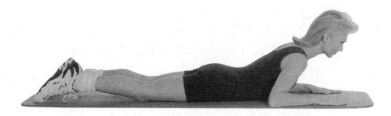

STARTING POSITION   Lie on your stomach with your hands by your head, elbows bent at right angles and forearms on the floor, head down.

ACTION   Exhale as you press up with your hands so you're arching your back slightly, but still looking down. Hold for three counts, then inhale as you release. Repeat ten times.

Benefits erector spinae and lower back

(Since this exercise is more advanced, you may want to build up your strength before doing it. If you're not ready, you can proceed to the Flexibility Cooldown.)

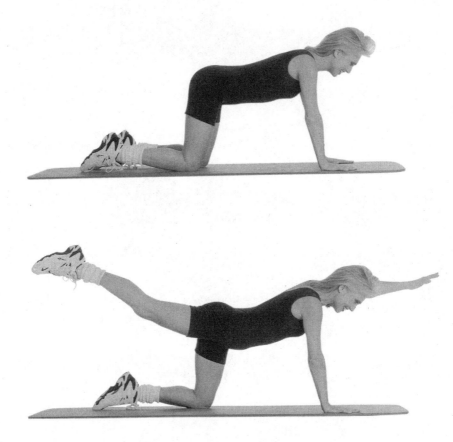

STARTING POSITION   Start on your hands and knees, facedown.

ACTION   Exhale as you extend and lift your left arm and right leg. Remain facedown as you hold for three seconds, inhale, and lower. Repeat ten times, alternating sides.

FLEXIBILITY COOLDOWN

Hold each stretch for ten to thirty seconds.

QUADRICEP STRETCH Lie on your stomach, facedown. Bend your right knee behind you and grab hold of your foot. Bring your heel toward your buttocks, as close as possible without straining, breathing deeply. Slowly release down. Repeat with left leg.

HAMSTRING STRETCH Turn onto your back. Bend both knees and place your feet flat on the floor. Bend your right knee in to your chest, then extend the leg straight up, keeping both hips on the floor. If you want additional stretch, you can wrap both hands around your thigh and gently pull the leg in toward your body. Release by bending your knee, then lowering it to the floor. Repeat with left leg.

CHEST STRETCH Roll onto one side, then use your hands to help yourself up to standing, gently and slowly. Go into a doorway and hold on to the sides with your elbows bent at 90-degree angles. Step forward with one leg, as if you're walking into the room, so that your elbows are slightly behind you and your chest is open. Hold and breathe into the stretch, then gently release.

NECK AND SHOULDER STRETCH Stand tall, then tilt your head to the left side and the right. Extend your right arm up and stretch; then stretch your left arm. Roll your shoulders back a few times. Shake out any spots that feel tight.

LIFESTYLE LIFTS

GET YOUR OPTIMAL DAILY AMOUNT OF CALCIUM The week you begin the 4-Week Workout Program is a good time to look at your daily calcium intake. Determine if it measures up to the optimal dosage recommendations, which are:

- 1,000 mg daily for premenopausal women and those who take estrogen
- 1,500 mg daily for menopausal and postmenopausal women who do not take estrogen

If you need more calcium, review the lists of calcium-rich foods in Chapter 11 and plan how to increase your consumption. Food sources of calcium are the most desirable, but if you're not sure you can consume enough calcium on a daily basis, you can also take high-quality supplements.

Since vitamin D is necessary for calcium absorption, be sure to take in 400 IU of this nutrient each day. If you don't get out in the sunlight on a daily basis, you may want to take a multivitamin supplement that includes D.

During the month of the Workout Program, keep a daily record of your calcium consumption. By the end of four weeks, you should be familiar with the calcium content of foods and accustomed to getting enough of this vital mineral every day.

ESTABLISH HEALTHY POSTURAL HABITS

Good posture is crucial for women with osteoporosis, to avoid additional stress on the spine. If you become conscious of maintaining healthy body mechanics in everyday activities, it will help prevent strain, falls, and fractures. The following postural ideas will help you avoid injury.

▸ Use a pillow or a rolled towel as a support behind your lower back in soft couches and chairs or bucket seats in cars.

▸ Try to use the headrest in the car to support your neck.

▸ When reading, hold the material up instead of looking down at it.

▸ When working at a desk, be aware of your posture and try to maintain the natural curve of your spine. Work in a well-designed office chair, or use towels and small pillows as supports if necessary. Use a clipboard or a typing stand to hold up material you're reading or typing.

▸ Hold the phone up to your ear instead of jamming it between your head and shoulder. If you're on the phone a great deal, consider purchasing a telephone headset.

▸ When standing, keep your shoulders down and back. Maintain the natural curve of your spine. If you need to stand for a long time, alternate putting one foot and then the other up on a small stool, step, or open cupboard.

▸ Whether you're doing everyday activities, lifting, or exercising, always avoid bending from the waist. When moving to the floor, go down on one knee while your hands are on top of the opposite thigh.

▸ Avoid twisting movements, whether in an exercise class or during daily activities such as cleaning or yard work.

▸ When getting into bed, first sit down on the side of the bed. Lie down on your side, bringing your feet onto the bed one at a time. Take a breath as you roll onto your back with your knees bent and arms in front of you. To get out of bed, reverse this action: first roll onto your side. Use your hands to raise your body as you gently put both legs over the side of the bed. Sit on the edge and relax for a minute, then get up slowly to avoid dizziness.

ACCIDENT PREVENTION Building your strength and stability through regular exercise will reduce your chance of falls and fractures. It's also helpful to accident-proof your environment as much as possible. Here are some hints:

- Avoid the use of small throw rugs. Secure all large rugs and runners on stairs.
- Have secure treads and handrails on your stairs.
- Remove any cables, cords, or other obstructions on the floor.
- Don't use slippery floor waxes or walk on wet floors.
- Install grab bars and nonskid tape in your shower/bath.
- Use a nonskid rubber mat near the stove and sink in the kitchen.
- Install good lighting in your hall, stairs, and entrances; use nightlights in the bedroom and bathroom.
- Use extra caution on wet and icy days outside. You shouldn't feel embarrassed to use a cane or hold a friend's arm for stability.
- Avoid high heels and backless slippers or sandals. Wear low-heeled, soft-soled shoes with good ankle and arch support.
- Continue doing the Workout for Women with Osteoporosis to feel stronger and more confident in all situations.

OTHER LIFESTYLE LIFTS You can also enjoy many of the Lifestyle Lifts described in Chapters 13–16. Read through these suggestions and choose the ones that appeal to you. Reward yourself with a spa treatment or healthy vacation to celebrate your fitness successes.

CHECKLIST FOR YOUR WORKOUT PROGRAM

‣ ‣

1. Discuss the aerobic and strength-training exercises you'll be doing in this program with your physician to confirm that they are safe for you.
2. Write down your exercise appointments: three to five sessions of aerobics and two of the strength routines.
3. Participate in an aerobic activity three to five times a week for thirty minutes or longer. (You may have to start with fifteen minutes at a time and build up to thirty.) Do the Warm-up and

Cooldown exercises before and after each aerobic session.

4. Perform the Strength Training Routine for Osteoporosis twice a week. Do the Warm-up and Cooldown exercises before and after each workout.

5. Increase your calcium intake to 1,000–1,500 mg per day, as much as possible through food sources. Also be sure to get 400 IU of vitamin D each day.

6. Become aware of your posture in your daily habits; make adjustments to avoid strain and injury.

7. Take steps to accident-proof your living environment.

8. Celebrate your success with a spa treatment or other Lifestyle Lifts.

9. Make a firm commitment to continue to exercise regularly and enjoy a healthier quality of life.

BETTER THAN EVER FOREVER

The expression "use it or lose it" is blunt but true. Fitness is an ongoing process. If you want to reduce the symptoms of menopause and the risk of osteoporosis and heart disease, you need to continue with a balanced, regular exercise program.

The goal is to be consistent. Each week, aim for at least three sessions of Aerobic Activity and two of strength training, with warm-up and cooldown stretching each time.

You can play with the pattern and do strength exercises on the same day as aerobics. For example, you might do twenty minutes on the treadmill or stair machine at the gym, followed by a weight workout. Or you can go for an aerobic walk outside, then do the Strength Training Routine at home.

STICKING WITH EXERCISE

There's no secret formula or absolute answer to the challenge of staying with an exercise program. But there are a few techniques I have found that work with my clients.

The first step is to write down your exercise appointments every week. Convince yourself that it's of paramount importance to keep these appointments since, in the long run, this is true.

Like a successful relationship, exercise takes commitment, desire, and willingness to work at it. If you need motivation, you can find it in the constant stream of articles and books about the effects of exercise on health, disease, and weight. You can also find inspiration in the people around you and the way you feel on a daily basis.

Pay attention to the difference in your energy level and mood when you exercise and when you don't. Add to that long-term concerns about heart disease, osteoporosis, and other conditions, and you have abundant reasons to continue. For more motivation, look in the mirror and think about the positive influence of exercise on posture, weight, body shape, and skin tone.

DEALING WITH SETBACKS

▶ ▶ ▶ ▶ ▶ ▶ ▶ ▶ ▶

Even with the best intentions there may be periods when you're not able to keep up with your exercise program. We're all human and life has its ups and downs. There are several ways you can deal with setbacks and get back on track.

If you find yourself missing exercise appointments on a regular basis, you may want to start the 4-Week Workout Program again and go through the week-by-week steps to give yourself structure. This can be a good way to get back in the swing and renew your commitment.

Another technique is to set workout dates with a close friend, someone who won't let you off the hook if you start making excuses. Or you can sign up for exercise classes, preferably with a teacher who knows you and will notice if you don't show up. You might also have a few sessions with a personal trainer to get the ball rolling.

If you have a setback period, don't waste your time blaming yourself, feeling guilty, or debating whether or not to work out. Give your mind a rest and let your body take over.

Do some work around your home to wake up your muscles. Take a walk outside or dance to some music you love. Once you've shaken off your lethargy, you'll have more energy to return to your exercise program.

Keep in mind that no matter what mood you're in, you'll feel better after you exercise. I have never once heard anyone say, "Gee, I wish I didn't do that, I really feel worse now," after a workout. But hundreds of times I've heard women say, "I didn't feel like exercising, but I'm glad I did." Trust that feeling and go for it.

PROGRESSING IN YOUR AEROBIC EXERCISE

▶ ▶ ▶ ▶ ▶ ▶ ▶ ▶ ▶

After two months of doing aerobic exercise at least three times a week, you may be ready to increase the challenge. The safest way to start is by increasing the duration and frequency of your aerobic workouts, rather than the intensity. This principle can be used by women at all fitness levels and by those with osteoporosis.

Add five and then ten minutes to your sessions. Check your heart rate to see if you're still in your THR zone. In another month, add five or ten more minutes. Check your pulse again to see if you're working in your THR zone. If you're doing well and staying within your range, you can continue to add to the duration. Always be sensitive to how you feel and to the weather conditions, and reduce the time if you experience any discomfort or injuries.

After three months of exercising aerobically, you may want to play around with the intensity. You can do this by increasing your heart rate for a few minutes, but not extending beyond your THR zone. For example, if you're walking, you might go up a steep hill; if you're biking, do a little sprint. If you have osteoporosis, you need to be sensible when increasing the intensity.

Another way to progress in aerobics is to work out four or five days a week instead of three. Some people like to do aerobics six days a week, which is fine if you do cross training—varying the workout by changing the type, duration, or intensity—to reduce the risk of overuse injury.

After three or four months, you may want to retake the walk/run test in Chapter 6 and reassess your fitness level. If you've moved into a higher level, you can start on more challenging activities; for example, jogging instead of walking, or advanced step classes.

BUILDING ON THE STRENGTH TRAINING ROUTINE

▶ ▶ ▶ ▶ ▶ ▶ ▶ ▶ ▶ ▶

After you've completed the first four weeks of the program, repeat the Strength Training Routines sequentially for the next month. You can follow this pattern:

WEEK 5:	Repeat Week 1 routine
WEEK 6:	Repeat Week 2 routine
WEEK 7:	Repeat Week 3 routine
WEEK 8:	Repeat Week 4 routine

If you do the special workout for women with osteoporosis, continue with the same routine for the second month. Then you can begin to modify the routine by adding to your sets, reps, or weights.

After doing the workouts for two months, twice a week, you're likely to find your strength level changing and the exercises becoming easier. When you feel this way it's time to modify the routines. Here are options for progressing in the strength workouts:

1. Review the fitness tests in Chapter 6. If you've reached a higher level by those criteria, do those exercises at your new level for each Strength Training Routine.

2. Increase the number of repetitions. For instance, Level 1 can progress to one set of twelve. The number of repetitions caps at fifteen.
3. Increase the number of sets. For example, Level 1 can progress to two sets of eight. The number of sets caps at three.
4. Increase the amount of weight lifted.
5. Add another day or two of your strength routines.

You can continue to do the four workouts sequentially each month with these various modifications. A bonus is that you'll learn the exercises by heart. You can check the list of exercises at the end of this chapter and perform them without reading through the instructions. Every two months or so you can reassess your fitness level and increase the challenge in one of the five ways.

If you're adding weights, you'll probably reach a plateau at 10–12 lbs. for hand weights and 5 lbs. for ankle weights. Eventually, you'll also reach a plateau with your sets and reps. At that point you can continue to do the workouts at your peak level to maintain your muscle and bone strength. If you want to get into more serious muscle building or body sculpting, you can join a gym with various equipment and qualified instructors.

STAYING ACTIVE AND FIT

▶ ▶ ▶ ▶ ▶ ▶ ▶ ▶ ▶ ▶

Remember that there's more to fitness than structured workouts. Stretching, relaxation practices, and nutrition are also key to your well-being. Take the time to nurture every aspect of your body and mind. You deserve it. You'll be a happier person and the people around you will also benefit.

If you find yourself getting bored with your exercise program, the solution is simple: Do something different or increase the challenge.

Set mini-goals for yourself. For instance, you can join a "Y" or club that has a pool and set a goal of doing fifty laps by the end of the summer. Participate in a 5k run, even if you need to walk most of the course. Bike to a friend's house instead of driving. Join a walkathon or bikeathon for your favorite cause. These challenges can be rewarding.

Be adventurous and creative in your exercise life. Go snorkeling on a beach vacation. Sign up for a hiking expedition or canoe trip. Take an exotic dance class. Follow your pleasure and expand your limits.

If you stay active and fit, midlife can be the most vital and satisfying time of your life. You can experience more independence, success, and stability than ever before. Exercise can give you the confidence, energy, and ability to enjoy all life has to offer.

THE 4-WEEK WORKOUT PROGRAM: STRENGTH TRAINING ROUTINE

▶ ▶ ▶ ▶ ▶ ▶ ▶ ▶ ▶ ▶ ▶ ▶ ▶ ▶ ▶ ▶ ▶ ▶ ▶ ▶

WEEK 1

Warm-up

1. One-arm Row
2. Leg Extensions
3. Wrist Curls—Palms Up
4. Wrist Curls—Palms Down
5. Leg Curls
6. Standing Wall Pushup/Modified Pushup
7. Wing-out
8. Pelvic Tilt with Kegels
9. Curl-ups
10. Reverse Curls
11. Twists
12. Alternating Arm/Leg Lift
13. Press-ups I
14. Alternating Push

Flexibility Cooldown

WEEK 2

Warm-up

1. Chest Press
2. Outer Thigh Leg Lifts
3. Inner Thigh Leg Lifts
4. Bicep Curls
5. Overhead Press
6. Tricep Kickbacks
7. Pelvic Tilt with Kegels
8. Curl-ups
9. Double Bent-knee Lift
10. Bicycles
11. Press-ups I
12. Alternating Push
13. All Fours Alternating Arm/Leg Lift

Flexibility Cooldown

WEEK 3

Warm-up

1. Wall Pushup with Triangle/Modified Pushup
2. One-arm Row
3. Angled Outer Thigh Lifts
4. Inner Thigh Pulse Lifts
5. Wing-out
6. Pelvic Tilt with Kegels
7. Curl-ups with Pulses
8. Baby Bicycles
9. Bicycles
10. Press-ups I
11. Press-ups II
12. All Fours Alternating Arm/Leg Lift

Flexibility Cooldown

WEEK 4

Warm-up

1. Wall Slide
2. Concentrated Bicep Curls
3. Wrist Curls—Palms Up
4. Wrist Curls—Palms Down
5. Dips
6. Lateral Raises
7. Pelvic Tilt with Kegels
8. Curl-ups
9. Reverse Curls
10. Twists
11. Press-ups II
12. All Fours Alternating Arm/Leg Lift
13. Arm Circles

Flexibility Cooldown

WORKOUT FOR WOMEN WITH OSTEOPOROSIS

▶ ▶ ▶ ▶ ▶ ▶ ▶ ▶ ▶ ▶ ▶ ▶ ▶ ▶ ▶ ▶ ▶ ▶ ▶

Warm-up

1. Standing Wall Pushup
2. Leg Curls
3. Press-backs
4. Leg Extensions
5. Bicep Curls
6. Wrist Curls—Palms Up
7. Wrist Curls—Palms Down
8. Pelvic Tilt with Kegels

9. Single-leg Slide
10. Single Bent-knee Lift
11. Bent-knee Lift with Opposite-leg Slide
12. Alternating Arm Lift
13. Alternating Leg Lift
14. Alternating Arm/Leg Lift
15. Press-ups I
16. All Fours Alternating Arm/Leg Lift (Advanced)

Flexibility Cooldown

SUGGESTED READING AND RESOURCES

Bailey, Covert, and Lea Bishop, *The Fit or Fat Woman*. Boston: Houghton Mifflin, 1989.

Benson, Herbert, M.D., *The Mind/Body Effect*. New York: Berkeley Books, 1979.

Budoff, Penny Wise, M.D., *No More Hot Flashes, and Other Good News*. New York: Warner Books, revised 1989.

Clark, Nancy, M.S., R.D., *Nancy Clark's Sports Nutrition Guidebook*. Champaign, IL: Leisure Press, 1990.

Cone, Faye Kitchener, *Making Sense of Menopause*. New York: Fireside/Simon & Schuster, 1993.

Cooper, Kenneth H., *The New Aerobics for Women*. New York: Bantam Books, 1988.

Cutler, Winifred, B., Ph.D., and Celso-Ramon Garcia, M.D., *Menopause, A Guide for Women and the Men Who Love Them*. New York: W. W. Norton, 1992.

Evans, William, Ph.D., and Irwin H. Rosenberg, M.D., with Jacqueline Thompson, *Biomarkers: The 10 Keys to Prolonging Vitality*. New York: Fireside/Simon & Schuster, 1992.

Gillespie, Clark, M.D., *Hormones, Hot Flashes and Mood Swings*. New York: Harper & Row, 1994.

Greenwood, Sadja, M.D., *Menopause Naturally*. Volcano, CA: Volcano Press, 1992.

Jacobowitz, Ruth S., *150 Most-Asked Questions About Menopause*. New York: Hearst Books, 1993.

Lark, Susan M., M.D., *The Menopause Self-Help Book*. Berkeley, CA: Celestial Arts, 1990.

Legato, Marianne, M.D., and Carol Colman, *The Female Heart: The Truth About Women and Heart Disease*. New York: Avon Books, 1991.

Melpomene Institute for Women's Health Resources, *The Bodywise Woman*. New York: Prentice Hall, 1990.

Nachtigall, Lila, M.D., and Joan Rattner Heilman, *Estrogen: The Facts Can Change Your Life*. New York: HarperCollins, 1991.

Notelovitz, Morris, M.D., Ph.D., and Diana Tonnessen, *Menopause and Midlife Health*. New York: St. Martin's Press, 1994.

Ornish, Dean, M.D., *Dr. Ornish's Program for Reversing Heart Disease*. New York: Random House, 1990.

Peck, William A., M.D., and Louis Avioli, M.D., *Osteoporosis—the Silent Thief*. Glenview, IL: AARP Books, 1988.

Sheehy, Gail, *The Silent Passage*. New York: Pocket Books, 1993.

Utian, Wulf H., M.D., Ph.D., and Ruth S. Jacobowitz, *Managing Your Menopause*. New York: Fireside/Simon & Schuster, 1990.

Whitaker, Julian M., M.D., *Reversing Heart Disease*. New York: Warner Books, 1985.

FYI
▸ ▸ ▸ ▸ ▸ ▸ ▸ ▸ ▸ ▸

A *Friend Indeed*, a monthly newsletter addressing all issues of midlife women, by Janine O'Leary Cobb. P.O. Box 1710, Champlain, NY 12919; (514) 843-5730.

Hadassah, the Women's Zionist Organization of America, Inc., Health Education Department, 50 West 58th Street, New York, NY 10019.

Lisa Hoffman, M.A., Solo Fitness, P.O. Box 1526, Madison Square Station, New York, NY 10010; e-mail: Solofitness@compuserve.com.

The Melpomene Institute, a nonprofit organization dedicated to bringing together physical activity and health through education, research, and publications. 1010 University Avenue, St. Paul, MN 55104; (612) 642-1951.

National Coalition for Women in Midlife, 327 Central Park West, New York, NY 10025; (212) 666-6579.

National Osteoporosis Foundation, 1150 17th St. N.W., Suite 500, Washington, D.C. 20036; (800) 223-9994 or (202) 223-2226.

North American Menopause Society, P.O. Box 94527, Cleveland, OH 44101-4527; (900) 370-NAMS (6267).

CHAPTER NOTES

CHAPTER 1 Ruth S. Jacobowitz, *150 Most-Asked Questions About Menopause* (New York: Hearst Books, 1993): p. 33.

Ibid., p. 55.

Emrika Padus, *Your Emotions & Your Health* (Emmaus, PA: Rodale Press, 1986), p. 94.

Cathy Perlmutter with Toby Hanlong and Maureen Sangiorno, "Triumph Over Menopause," *Prevention* 46, No. 8 (August 1994): 80–87.

CHAPTER 2 Mats Hammer, Goran Berg, and Richard Lindgren, "Does Physical Exercise Influence the Frequency of Postmenopausal Hot Flushes?" *Acta Obstet Gynecol Scand* 69 (1990): 409–12.

CHAPTER 4 Gail Dalksy, Ph.D., et al., "Weight-Bearing Exercise Training and Lumbar Bone Mineral Content in Postmenopausal Women," *Annals of Internal Medicine* 108 (1988): 201–4.

"FDA Advisory Committee Recommends Approval of New Osteoporosis Drug," *Osteoporosis Report*, National Osteoporosis Foundation, Vol. II, no. 2/Summer 1995.

Miriam E. Nelson, Ph.D., et al., "Effects of High-Intensity Strength Training on Multiple Risk Factors for Osteoporotic Fractures," *Journal of the American Medical Association* 272 (December, 1994): 1909–14.

Beth Anne Piper, M.D., Theresa D. Galsworthy, R.N., Richard S. Bockman, M.D., Ph.D.; Diagnosis and Management of Osteoporosis," *Contemporary Internal Medicine*, July 1995.

"Update: Bisphosphonates; Update: Fluoride," *Lunar News*, Lunar Corporation, December 1995.

CHAPTER 5   Jane E. Brody, "Personal Health," *New York Times*, (November 10, 1993): p. C17.

Jane E. Brody, "Personal Health," *New York Times*, (February 8, 1995): p. C17.

Ruth Jacobowitz, *150 Most-Asked Questions About Menopause* (New York: Hearst Books, 1993), p. 135.

Marianne J. Legato, M.D., "Managing Heart Disease Risk in Post-menopausal Women," *The Female Patient*, AMA/CME 18 (April 1993): 33–43.

CHAPTER 6   Borg, G. A. V., "Psychological Bases of Physical Exertion," *Medicine and Science in Sport and Exercise*, ACSM 14 (1982): 377–87.

William Evans, Ph.D., Irwin H. Rosenberg, M.D., with Jacqueline Thompson, *Biomarkers: The 10 Keys to Prolonging Longevity* (New York: Simon & Schuster, 1991), pp. 53–60.

CHAPTER 9   Jane E. Brody, "Personal Health," *New York Times*, (August 10, 1994): p. C8.

Evans and Rosenberg, *Biomarkers*, pp. 42–47.

Michelle Nicolosi, "Pumping Up," *Shape Magazine* (Winter, 1994): 64.

CHAPTER 10   Herbert Benson, M.D., with Miriam Z. Klipper, *The Relaxation Response* (New York: Avon Books, 1975), pp. 158–74.

Berkeley Holistic Health Center, *Holistic Health Lifebook* (Lexington, MA: The Stephen Greene Press, 1985), pp. 127–33.

Leonard M. Germaine, M.D., and Robert R. Freedman, M.D., "Behavior and Treatment of Menopausal Hot Flashes," *Journal of Consulting and Clinical Psychology* 52 (1984): 1072–79.

CHAPTER 11   Shari Lieberman, Ph.D., C.N.S., "On Nutrition and Health," *New Life* (March/April, 1995): p. 25.

Mindell, Earl, *Earl Mindell's Vitamin Bible* (New York: Warner Books, 1979), p. 72.

Ibid., p. 38.

National Osteoporosis Foundation, *Physician's Resource Manual on Osteoporosis: A Decision-Making Guide*, Second Edition (NOF, 1991).

National Research Council, *Recommended Dietary Allowance*, Tenth Edition (Washington, D.C.: National Academy Press, 1989).

Molly O'Neill, "So It May Be True After All: Eating Pasta Makes You Fat," *New York Times* (February 6, 1995), p. 1.

Ibid., p. C6.

ADDITIONAL SOURCES

ACSM's Guidelines for Exercise Testing and Prescription, 5th ed. Media, PA: Williams & Wilkins, 1995.

Boning Up on Osteoporosis, a publication of the National Osteoporosis Center, University of Connecticut Health Center, 1991.

Menopause: The Journal of the North American Menopause Society, 1994, 1995.

More Facts You Need to Know, a publication of the National Osteoporosis Information Center, Washington, D.C., 1994.

William D. McCardle, Frank I. Katch, and Victor L. Katch, *Exercise Physiology: Energy, Nutrition, and Human Performance*, 3rd ed. Malvern, PA: Lea & Febiger, 1991.

Mona Shangold, M.D., and Gabe Mirkin, M.D., *Women and Exercise Physiology and Sports Medicine*, 2nd ed. Philadelphia: F.A. Davis Co., 1994.

Wulf Utian, M.D., Ph.D., et al., "A Consensus Opinion, Calcium Supplementation for the Prevention and Treatment of Osteoporosis," *Menopause Management*, May/June, 1994: pp. 1–13.

INDEX

for women with osteoporosis,
171–86
Strength tests, 29
Strength training, 36
benefits of, 53–54
building on, 193–194
definition, 56
fat loss and muscle building,
54–55
importance for midlife women,
53–54
types, 56–57
Strength Training Routines, 36,
57–58
Stress, 23
and exercise, 3–4
physiological responses to,
63–64
Stretching, 36–37
benefits of, 60–61
breaks, 62–63
and flexibility, 60
safe ways of, 61–62
women with osteoporosis and,
62
Swimming, 39, 40, 47–48, 52

Target Heart Rate zone, 29–31, 42,
128
Tennis, 46–47
Tests
aerobic, 28
bone density, 15–16
strength, 29
Thompson, Jacqueline, 54
THR zone. *See* Target Heart Rate
zone
Thyroid hormones, 15
Treadmills, 43
Tricep Kickbacks, 116
Twists, 102, 159

USDA Human Nutrition
Research Center on Aging,
17, 54

Vitamin D
and calcium absorption, 77
intake for women with osteoporosis, 188
and maintaining bone density,
74
and osteoporosis prevention, 74
Vliet, Elizabeth Lee, 1, 60
Volleyball, 47

Walking, 39, 40–41, 51, 52
Wall pushups, 95
Wall pushups, with triangle, 13
Wall slides, 149
Warm-up exercises
week 1 of 4-Week Workout Pro-
gram, 88–89
week 2 of 4-Week Workout Pro-
gram, 110
week 3 of 4-Week Workout Pro-
gram, 129
week 4 of 4-Week Workout Pro-
gram, 148
for women with osteoporosis,
170
Warning signs, 26–27
Water, 71–72, 107
Weight, 8–10
Weight-bearing exercise, xiv, 17,
18, 39–40
Weightlifting, 54, 58–59
Weights, 85
Whitaker, Julian, 24
Wing-outs, 97, 135
Wolff's Law, 16–17
Women with osteoporosis
accident prevention, 189

aerobic exercises for, 168–69
arm lifts, 182
arm/leg lifts, 184, 186
bent-knee lifts, 180, 181
biking, 48–49
calcium intake, 187–88
checklist for Workout Program,
189–90
cooldown stretching exercises,
187
exercise guidelines, 18
finding fitness level, 29
4-Week Workout Program, 86
high-impact aerobic exercises,
46–47
Kegel exercises for, 178
posture habits, 188–89
rowing, 49–50
stretching and, 62
swimming, 47–48
vitamin D intake, 188
Workout Program for
checklist for, 189–90
cooldown stretching
exercises, 187
lifestyle lifts for, 187–89
strength exercises,
171–86
warm-up exercises, 170
wrist curls, 176, 177
Workout buddies, 85–86
Workout clothing, 84–85
World Health Organization, 16
Wrist curls
palms down, 93, 152
palms up, 92, 151
women with osteoporosis, 176,
177

Yoga, 68
Yoga breathing, 65

$$\frac{12)}{60}$$